COLOUR ATLAS OF PAEDIATRIC DERMATOLOGY

COLOUR ATLAS OF PAEDIATRIC DERMATOLOGY

Julian Verbov

MD (Liverpool), FRCP (London), MIBiol (London)
Consultant Dermatologist
Royal Liverpool Children's Hospital
England

Neil Morley

MB (Edinburgh), FRCP (Edinburgh), FRCP (Glasgow)
Consultant Dermatologist
Royal Hospital for Sick Children
Glasgow, Scotland

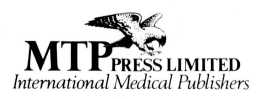

MTP PRESS LIMITED
International Medical Publishers

Published in the UK and Europe by
MTP Press Limited
Falcon House
Lancaster, England

British Library Cataloguing in Publication Data

Verbov, Julian
    Colour atlas of paediatric dermatology
    1. Pediatric dermatology
    I. Title   II. Morley, Neil
    618.92′5   RJ511

    ISBN 0–85200–474–5

Printed by Mather Bros (Printers) Limited
Preston, England

Contents

	Acknowledgements	7
	Preface	9
Chapter 1	Developmental abnormalities	10
Chapter 2	Genodermatoses	26
Chapter 3	The newborn	40
Chapter 4	Atopic and other types of dermatitis	56
Chapter 5	Infections and infestations	70
Chapter 6	Psoriasis and other erythemato-squamous disorders	88
Chapter 7	Vascular disorders	98
Chapter 8	Connective tissue disorders	110
Chapter 9	Bullous dermatoses	118
Chapter 10	Hair and nails	126
Chapter 11	Trauma, drug eruptions, and miscellaneous	138
	Index	154

Acknowledgements

We are indebted to Mrs A. F. Pearcey of the Royal Liverpool Hospital Department of Medical Illustration, Mr I. McKie of the Department of Dermatology, Western Infirmary, Glasgow, Mr J. Devlin of the Department of Medical Illustration, Royal Hospital for Sick Children, Glasgow, and Mr G. Hotchkiss of the Department of Pathology, Noble's Isle of Man Hospital, for providing and allowing reproduction of some of the photographs in this book, copyright of which remains with the aforementioned institutions.

We should like to thank the many colleagues who have allowed us to use photographs of their patients.

Finally we should like to thank Mrs Hazel Verbov for her painstaking efforts in typing and retyping the manuscript.

Preface

We have felt for some years that an atlas of paediatric dermatology merited a place in the world dermatological literature. Non-dermatologists find skin conditions difficult to describe and diagnose and this may be even more difficult in children. We usually rely on the parents for a history in children, although many conditions can be spot diagnoses.

In this atlas we have tried to illustrate conditions seen regularly in our clinics as well as some seen more rarely but which are nevertheless important to recognize. We have limited the number of illustrations in order to produce a realistically-priced book and thus it has not always been easy to decide what to include and what to omit. However, we hope that we have produced a reasonably comprehensive work.

We hope that this atlas will have a wide appeal both at home and abroad. It is a book either to read or to browse through. It is intended for senior medical students, family practitioners, and for trainees both in dermatology and in paediatrics. We would like it actually taken to skin clinics to be available for instant perusal, and to be on hand in the paediatric ward. We have said comparatively little about treatment because this alters regularly and often varies in different centres and because we do not think that an atlas is the place for this.

Julian Verbov

Neil Morley

1
Developmental abnormalities

SUPERNUMERARY NIPPLE (Figure 1.1)

Supernumerary nipples usually develop along the course of the embryological milk lines, which run from the anterior axillary folds to the inner thighs. They occur in both sexes. They can be confused with pigmented naevi or viral warts if not considered as a possibility.

AURICULAR APPENDAGE (Figure 1.2)

An auricular appendage or tag arises as a result of the development of accessory annular hillocks during the development of the external ear. They appear as fleshy nodules anterior to the ear.

CONGENITAL LYMPHOEDEMA (Figure 1.3)

Lymphoedema indicates diffuse soft-tissue swelling caused by accumulation of lymph due to inadequate lymphatic drainage. In congenital lymphoedema the area involved is swollen at birth. The swelling is firm and pits on pressure. When occurring in females and if hypoplastic toenails are present Turner's syndrome should be suspected.

PIGMENTED NAEVI

Freckles (ephelides) (Figure 1.4) are light brown, well-defined macules which appear in early childhood rather than in infancy. There is no increase in the number of melanocytes in the pigmented macules but their melanosomes are long and rod-shaped. They occur especially on sun-exposed areas of skin in fair- or red-haired children and tend to fade in winter.

Café-au-lait patches (Figure 1.5) are hyperpigmented macules with well-defined borders and are usually of no pathological significance. However, six or more greater than 1·5 cm in diameter are presumptive evidence of neurofibromatosis. There is an increased incidence of these patches in tuberous sclerosis.

Mongolian patches (Figures 1.6, 1.7) are congenital macular slate-grey or black patches generally found over lumbosacral areas and buttocks but they can occur anywhere on

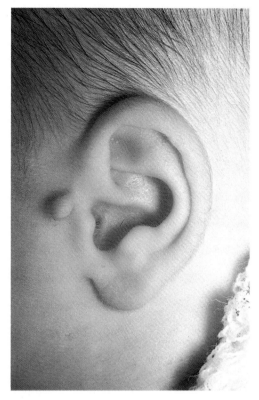

Figure 1.1 **Supernumerary nipple** inferior to right breast.

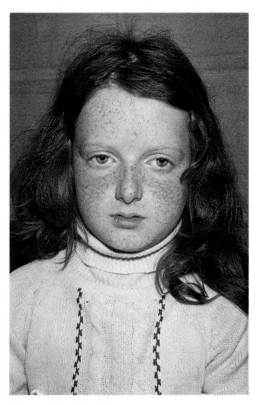

Figure 1.2 **Auricular appendage** anterior to pinna.

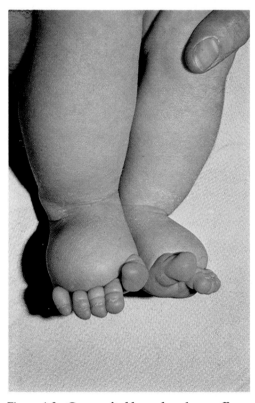

Figure 1.3 **Congenital lymphoedema** affecting lower legs in a 3-week-old male. He has gradually improved and was wearing normal shoes by the age of 3½ years. (Courtesy of Dr D. N. Williamson)

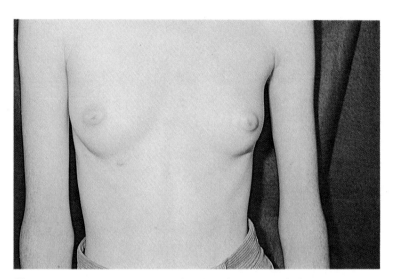

Figure 1.4 **Freckles.**

the skin including the face. Most negro and oriental babies show them but they are also present in less than 10% of caucasoids. They usually disappear by the end of the first decade. They represent collections of spindle-shaped melanocytes located deep in the dermis. It is important to distinguish them from bruises so as not to confuse them with non-accidental injury.

Blue naevus (Figures 1.8, 1.9) presents as a rounded area of blue or blue-black dermal pigmentation usually slightly raised and smooth-surfaced, produced by aberrant collections of functioning melanocytes. Common sites are dorsa of hands and feet, buttocks and face. Lesions may appear at birth or at any age. There are two types: the ordinary, and the less frequently seen cellular blue naevus which tends to be larger than 1 cm in diameter and which shows islands of large cells on histology not present in the ordinary blue naevus.

Melanocytic naevus (naevus–cell naevus) (Figure 1.10)

These lesions, often referred to as moles, are composed of naevus cells. They are divided into intradermal, junctional and compound, depending on the location of the cells. Thus, nests of naevus cells are situated solely in the dermis in intradermal naevi, at the junction of epidermis and dermis in junctional naevi, and both at the junction and in the dermis in compound naevi. Moles are very common, the majority appearing in childhood and adolescence. Face, neck and back are the usual sites and a very small fraction of the total become malignant, usually in adult life.

Intradermal naevi (Figure 1.11) are dome-shaped, sessile or pedunculated and may be non-pigmented or brown to black in colour. Coarse hairs are often present. They may occur anywhere on the skin surface and although usually small they can be greater than 1 cm in diameter.

Junctional naevi (Figure 1.12) are generally brown to black, hairless macules less than 1 cm in diameter. They often become compound naevi as the child ages.

Compound naevi (Figure 1.13) are seen in older children and tend to be more raised than junctional naevi. They may be hairy, particularly over the face. Clinically they may be indistinguishable from intradermal naevi.

Special forms of melanocytic naevus

Halo naevus (Sutton's naevus) (Figure 1.14) is a common lesion which presents usually over the trunk with a patch of depigmentation around a central, commonly melanocytic, naevus. Halo naevi may be single or multiple. The cause of the spontaneous depigmentation is unknown but there is an increased incidence of vitiligo in those with halo naevi. Lesions (halo and central lesion) have a tendency to spontaneous resolution.

Naevus spilus (Figure 1.15) is a solitary brown macule dotted with small brownish-black areas of pigmentation. It may vary from 1 to 20 cm in diameter and the histology is that of a dermal or junctional melanocytic naevus.

Giant pigmented naevus (Figure 1.16) presents at birth as an extensive pigmented hairy area often occupying the lower abdomen and buttocks to cover the bathing trunks area.

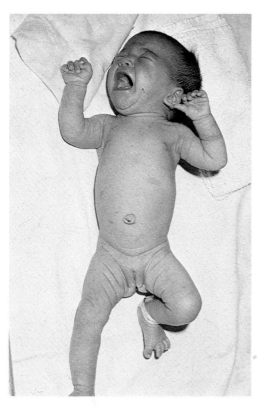

Figure 1.5 **Café-au-lait patches** (three are visible) over abdomen in a 6-week-old baby.

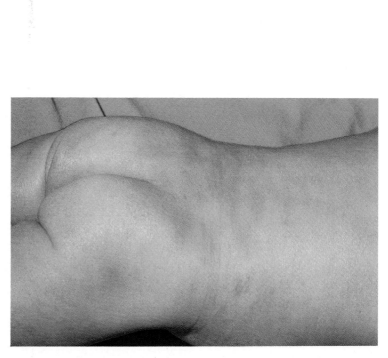

Figure 1.6 **Mongolian patches** in a Pakistani infant. Note the slaty-grey appearance of lesions.

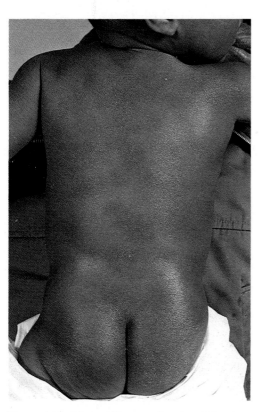

Figure 1.7 **Mongolian patches** in a Nigerian infant. Lesions have a blacker appearance in this darker-skinned child.

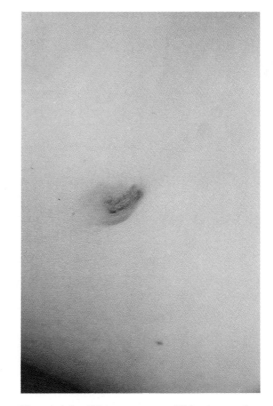

Figure 1.8 **Blue naevus** This shows the ordinary or common type.

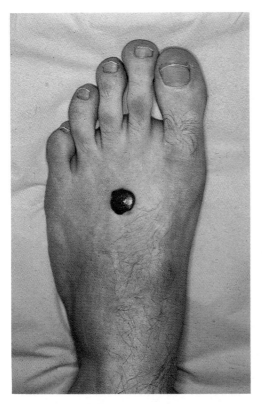

Figure 1.9   **Blue naevus**   This shows the less common cellular type. This lesion was excised because of suspicion of malignant melanoma but histology revealed its true and benign nature.

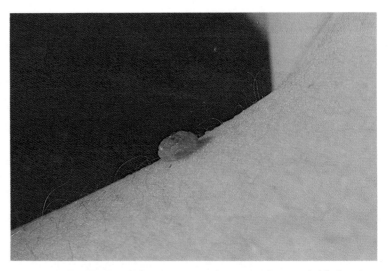

Figure 1.11   **Melanocytic naevus**   Close-up of same child showing dome-shaped sessile naevus over neck – intradermal naevus.

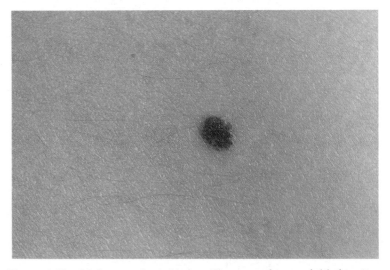

Figure 1.12   **Melanocytic naevus**   Close-up of same child showing dark-brown macular hairless naevus over right scapula – junctional naevus.

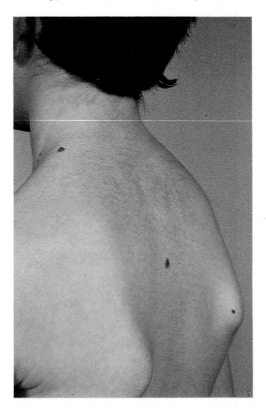

Figure 1.10   **Melanocytic naevus**   Child of 11 years showing three naevi.

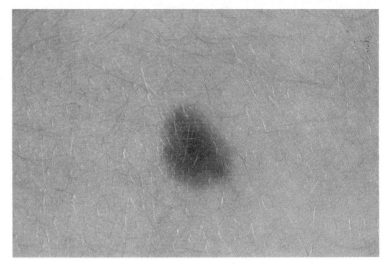

Figure 1.13   **Melanocytic naevus**   Close-up of same child showing interscapular slightly raised hairy naevus – compound naevus. It is likely to have developed from a purely junctional naevus.

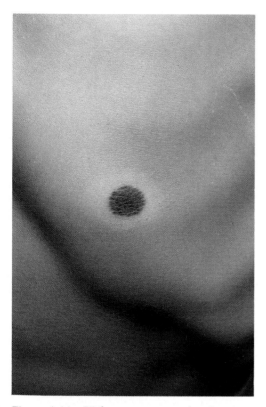

Figure 1.14 **Halo naevus** over the chest.

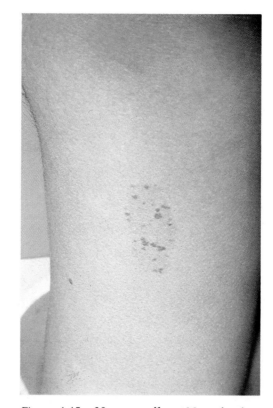

Figure 1.15 **Naevus spilus** Note the dots of darker pigmentation both at the edge and within the patch of pigmentation.

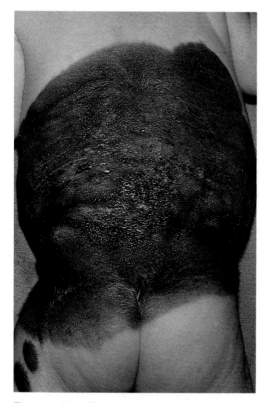

Figure 1.16 **Giant pigmented naevus** Extensive bathing trunks naevus in a 20-day-old child. A superficial erosion over the lower back present at birth healed spontaneously within a few days. She had many more smaller pigmented naevi scattered over the body. Now nearly 2 years old she has already had many lesions excised by plastic surgery.

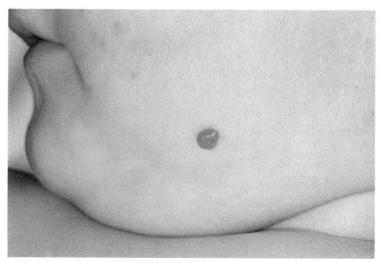

Figure 1.17 **Juvenile melanoma** Typical reddish-brown nodule.

They occur less frequently elsewhere. Treatment consists of surgical excision wherever possible because of the risk of malignant change in the large lesions. Facial lesions may require removal for cosmetic reasons.

Juvenile melanoma (spindle cell naevus) (Figures 1.17, 1.18)
This is a benign, usually solitary, tumour probably of melanocytic origin, which can occur anywhere on the skin surface. It presents as a firm smooth-surfaced dome-shaped nodule usually of reddish-brown colour correlated with the vascularity of the tumour, but it may be black and can have a warty appearance. Cells in the lesion are generally spindle-shaped, and multinucleated giant cells and mitotic figures are also present. The spindle and giant cells are two features distinguishing the lesion from malignant melanoma. The tumour can be excised.

DERMAL NAEVI
Haemangioma
Salmon patch (Figures 1.19, 1.20) is a common congenital, macular pink area indicating distended capillaries and situated over the forehead, glabella, upper eyelids and nape of neck. No treatment is necessary because lesions fade in the first year of life with the exception of the nuchal lesion (stork bite) which tends to persist but usually becomes covered by hair and thus unnoticed.

Port-wine stain (naevus flammeus) (Figures 1.21, 1.22) is always present at birth and is composed of irregularly dilated endothelial lined capillary vessels, confined to the upper dermis. They do not involute although some fade in colour slightly. They may, in fact, grow additional dilated vessels particularly over the face and these can bleed. Port-wine stains may occur at any skin site and there may be adjacent mucosal involvement. However, they are seen most commonly over head and neck. Those involving the supraorbital region are particularly likely to be associated with similar lesions involving the meninges on the same side, constituting the Sturge–Weber syndrome. Cosmetic cover is the recommended treatment for port-wine stains. Further development in laser therapy may make this a useful tool in some older children in the future.

Strawberry mark (superficial haemangioma) (Figures 1.23–1.27) is not usually present at birth but generally appears in the first month of life. Common sites are head, neck and trunk. They appear as well-defined small telangiectatic areas and grow to raised red lobulated tumours with capillaries visible over the surface. They grow rapidly with the child in the first year of life and then become stationary, involuting usually completely, over the next four or five years. Residual scarring may follow the occasional, often frictional lesion, that bleeds slightly, becomes infected, or ulcerates.

Cavernous haemangioma (Figures 1.28–1.30) can really be considered to be the same as a strawberry mark, only deeper. Lesions are composed of larger, mature vascular elements with involvement of both dermis and subcutaneous tissue. They are seen as bluish-red areas with indistinct borders. They do not grow as rapidly as strawberry marks. It is not uncommon for *mixed forms of strawberry and cavernous haemangioma* to occur. These lesions also resolve but resolution is not always complete. The rare Kasabach–Merritt syndrome, in which there is thrombocytopenia caused by platelet sequestration and destruction, occurs especially in giant cavernous haemangiomas.

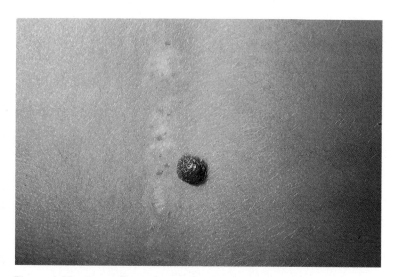

Figure 1.18 **Juvenile melanoma** Blacker lesion over the back near the midline.

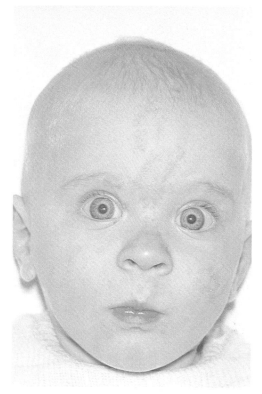

Figure 1.19 **Salmon patches** Typical pink patches over upper half of face which faded in the first year of life.

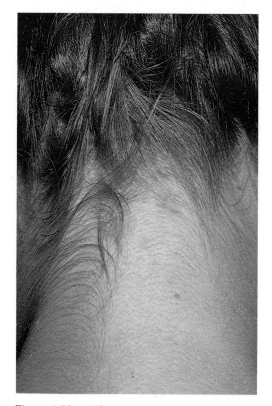

Figure 1.20 **Salmon patch** Girl of 15 with a nuchal patch; salmon patches at this site tend to persist.

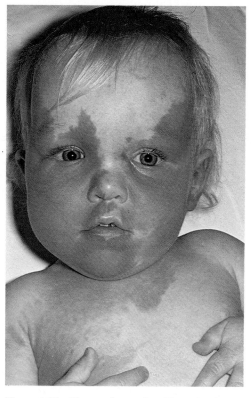

Figure 1.21 **Port-wine stain** Extensive lesion and these haemangiomata do not involve.

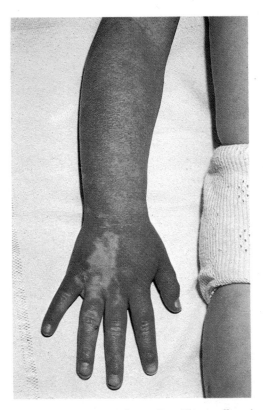

Figure 1.22 **Port–wine stain** The unaffected area of skin over the back of the hand shows up in contrast.

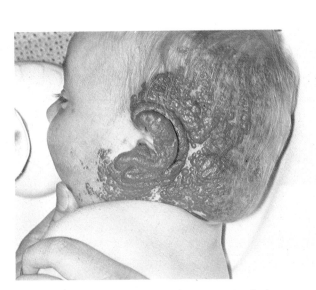

Figure 1.23 **Strawberry mark** Extensive lesion.

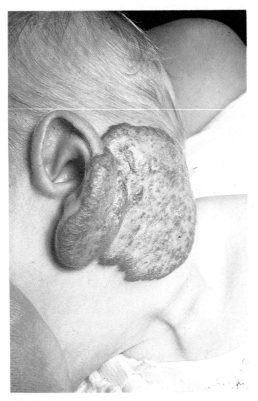

Figure 1.24 **Strawberry mark** Large hae-mangioma both behind and involving the pinna.

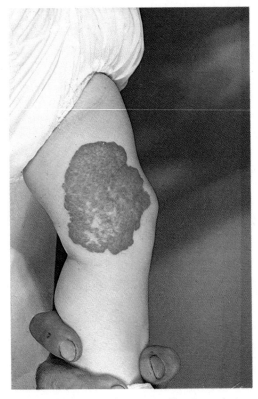

Figure 1.25 **Strawberry mark** Large lesion in a child 11 months old.

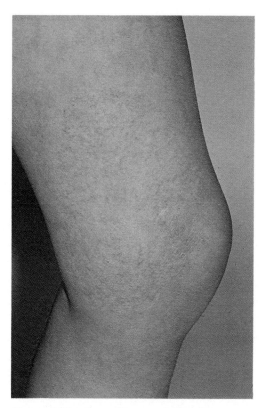

Figure 1.26 **Strawberry mark** Same area 5 years later.

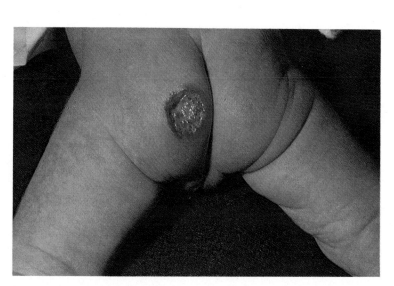

Figure 1.27 **Strawberry mark** Ulcerated lesion over buttock. Treated with topical antiseptics only.

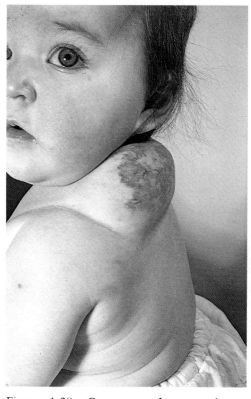

Figure 1.28 **Cavernous haemangioma** Large mainly cavernous haemangioma over back of neck.

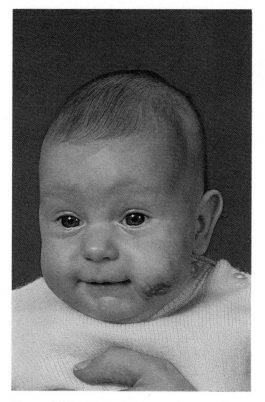

Figure 1.29 **Strawberry-cavernous haemangioma** Slight occasional bleeding of the strawberry element was easily controlled with gentle pressure.

Spider telangiectases (spider naevi) (Figure 1.31) consist of a central arteriole with radiating vessels. They are common and occur on the upper half of the body. Lesions occurring in healthy children tend to persist indefinitely. The central vessel can be destroyed with cautery or diathermy in the older child without any anaesthetic.

Angioma serpiginosum (Figure 1.32) is a rare disorder of the small dermal blood vessels and it occurs mainly in females. It usually has its onset in childhood and lower limbs and buttocks are the preferred sites. It begins as one or more small red or purple puncta which extend over a period of months or years. Lesions commonly follow the livedo patterning of the skin and there may be a background of diffuse erythema. Individual puncta may disappear and complete resolution may occur but is uncommon.

Lymphangioma circumscriptum (Figure 1.33) is the most common form of lymphangioma and presents at birth or in early childhood. It is characterized by groups of deep-seated thick-walled vesicles that simulate frog spawn. Frequently there is an haemangiomatous component. Common sites include proximal limbs, chest wall, and perineum.

Juvenile xanthogranuloma (Figure 1.34) is a self-limiting asymptomatic condition seen in infants and young children. It is much more common in whites than in negroes. Reddish single or multiple papules enlarge with the colour tending to yellow or brown. Histopathology reveals typical Touton giant cells which are histiocytes loaded with lipid. There is no evidence of abnormal lipid metabolism elsewhere and the lesions nearly always disappear before puberty.

EPITHELIAL NAEVI
Verrucous
Localized (Figure 1.35)

Lesions are usually solitary and are present at birth or appear in infancy or early childhood growing with the individual. They are skin-coloured or brown, raised with a rough warty surface. They vary in size and tend to be linear when over the limbs. Histopathology shows hyperkeratosis, papillomatosis, and acanthosis. If requiring treatment, excision by a plastic surgeon is recommended.

Widespread (naevus unius lateris) (Figures 1.36, 1.37)

In this naevus lesions are extensive and may form wavy transverse bands on the trunk and longitudinal, often spiral streaks on the limbs. Some of these naevi show histological features of epidermolytic hyperkeratosis (Chapter 2) and in some cases, may be a manifestation of that disorder.

Verrucous naevi, usually of the widespread type, may uncommonly be associated with developmental defects in other systems and such cases are referred to as the epidermal naevus syndrome.

Inflamed linear epidermal naevus (Figure 1.38) usually appears in infancy and is four times more common in females. It is pruritic and consists of scaly patches which appear as a linear eruption looking eczematous or psoriasiform in appearance. Most occur unilaterally over lower limb and buttock and may be very extensive. Histopathology reveals hyperkeratosis, parakeratosis, spongiosis and a dermal inflammatory infiltrate.

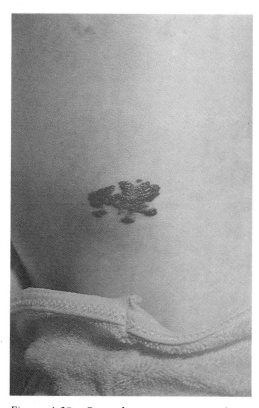

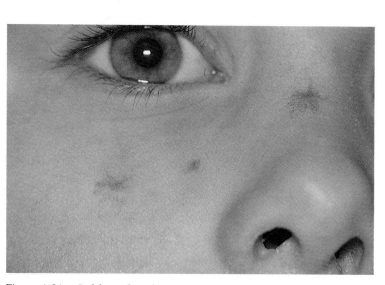

Figure 1.30 **Strawberry-cavernous hae-mangioma** This shows a mixed haemangioma on the trunk.

Figure 1.31 **Spider telangiectases** Three naevi can be seen each with a central arteriole.

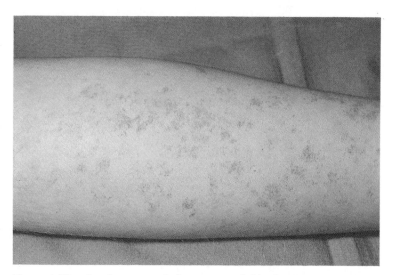

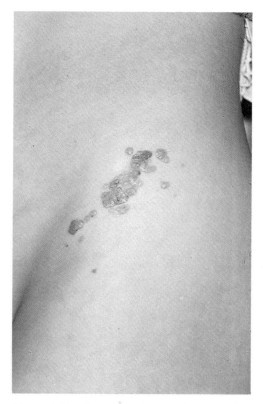

Figure 1.32 **Angioma serpiginosum** Child of 8 years showing the typical vascular puncta.

Figure 1.33 **Lymphangioma circumscriptum** Linear naevus over hip with an haemangiomatous element also.

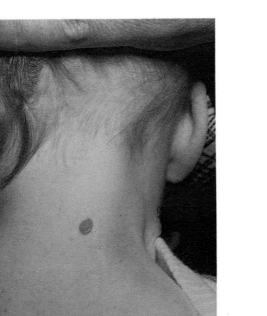

Figure 1.34 **Juvenile xanthogranuloma**
Solitary yellow-brown lesion over back of neck.

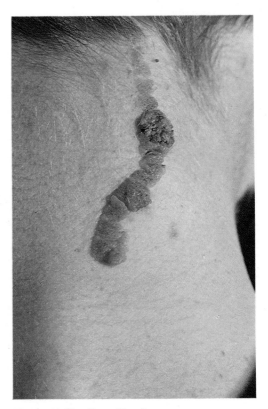

Figure 1.35 **Localized verrucous naevus**
Linear naevus localized to back of neck.

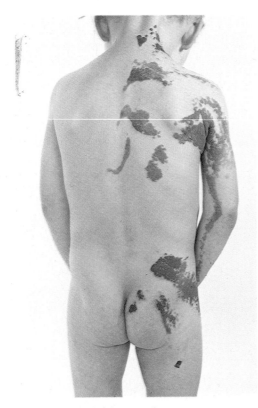

Figure 1.36 **Widespread verrucous naevus**
More extensive unilateral warty naevus.

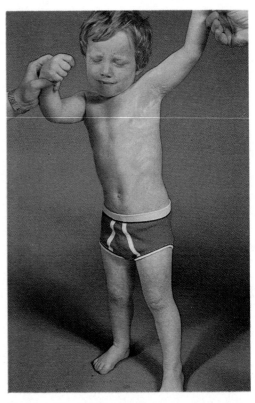

Figure 1.37 **Widespread verrucous naevus**
Wavy streaks of hyperkeratosis are visible over trunk. This child's lesions were not solely unilateral. The histopathology in some areas of a skin biopsy showed features of epidermolytic hyperkeratosis.

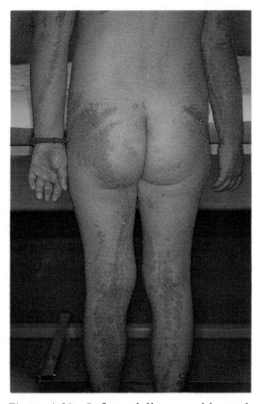

Figure 1.38 **Inflamed linear epidermal naevus** Bilateral mainly linear psoriasiform eruption in a 5-year-old girl. (Courtesy of Dr T. W. Stewart)

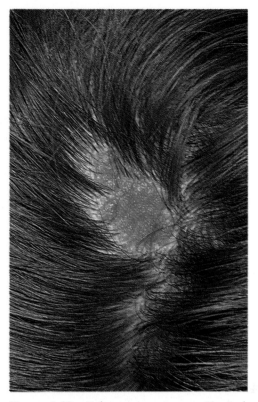

Figure 1.39 **Sebaceous naevus** Typical hairless scalp plaque with surface composed of closely packed rounded elevations.

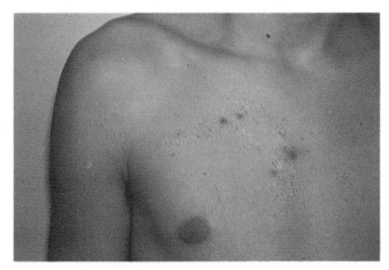

Figure 1.40 **Comedone naevus** Linear lesions over upper chest showing blackheads and folliculitis.

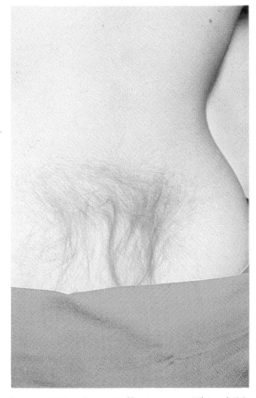

Figure 1.41 **Faun-tail naevus** This child had no defect underlying the excess hair.

Sebaceous naevus (Figure 1.39) is an uncommon but important congenital lesion containing both epidermal and dermal elements. Most common over the scalp they appear here as smooth, slightly raised, hairless waxy plaques, yellow-orange in colour and linear or somewhat oval in shape. Histologically there is an increase in the number of sebaceous glands which may also be enlarged and associated with hypertrophy and hyperkeratosis of the epidermis. Malignant transformation, particularly basal cell carcinoma, is not uncommon in these lesions and usually occurs from the fourth decade. Excision should be carried out in adolescence or early adult life as a precaution.

Comedone naevus (Figure 1.40)

Although sometimes present at birth this usually appears by the age of 20. The naevus consists of a group of dilated follicular orifices containing dark horny plugs. The area affected may be 2 cm in diameter or much more extensive. Face, neck, upper arm and chest are sites of predilection.

Faun-tail naevus (Figure 1.41)

Sometimes an abnormal growth of hair over the midline of the spine may indicate occult spina bifida. In view of the possible association of diastematomyelia with spina bifida the presence of any such lesions in children should lead to appropriate neurological referral.

2
Genodermatoses

Disease due to chromosomal abnormalities

DOWN'S SYNDROME (47, +21) has an incidence of around 1 in 600 live births. Although the skin is normal at birth it becomes increasingly dry with progressive age. Patients with Down's syndrome have an increased incidence of severe pyoderma. Alopecia areata occurs more frequently than in the general population and it tends to be extensive and persistent. The tongue is scrotal in almost all cases.

TURNER'S SYNDROME (Figure 2.1) (usually 45,X) affects 1 in 2500 live-born females. Infants may show lymphoedema of hands, feet and legs, and the nails may be hypoplastic. Older patients commonly show pigmented naevi, excessive keloid formation, and some skin hyperelasticity. Webbing of the neck is frequently present. The total finger ridge count is much higher than in individuals with XX sex chromosomal complement.

Disease due to single gene abnormalities

AUTOSOMAL DOMINANT
In this form of inheritance, on average half the offspring of an affected individual are also affected. However new mutations occur with a frequency which varies according to the condition.

Ectodermal dysplasia
Hidrotic ectodermal dysplasia (Figures 2.2, 2.3) is characterized by nail dystrophy, frequently associated with defects of hair and keratosis of palms and soles. Keratinization is abnormal and hyperkeratosis resulting from reduced desquamation is most evident over palms and soles. The nails are thickened, longitudinally striated, sometimes discoloured and grow slowly. Persistent paronychial infections are frequent and there is pebbly skin thickening beneath the free edges of the nails which fail to reach the tip of the digits.

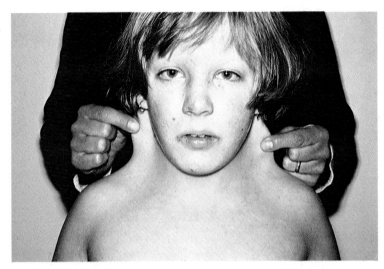

Figure 2.1 **Turner's syndrome** showing neck webbing. (Courtesy of Professor F. Harris)

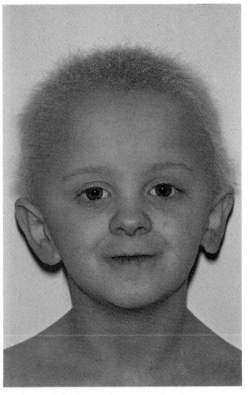

Figure 2.2 **Hidrotic ectodermal dysplasia** This 6½-year-old child had pale, brittle, scanty, fine hair.

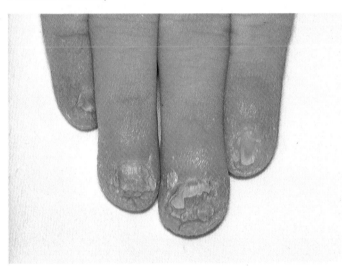

Figure 2.3 **Hidrotic ectodermal dysplasia** Child aged 5 showing pebbly skin thickening over finger tips. Short nails are also visible.

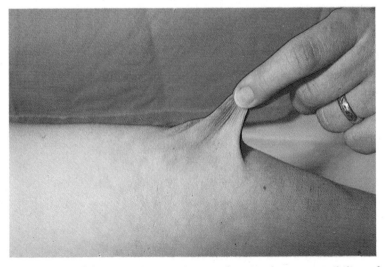

Figure 2.4 **Ehlers–Danlos syndrome** showing hyperextensibility of skin.

Sweating is normal and the facial appearance is normal but in the complete forms scalp hair is very sparse, fine, pale and brittle or even completely lacking.

Ehlers–Danlos syndrome (Figures 2.4–2.6) has at least eight clinically and genetically distinct variants all associated with abnormalities of collagen. The most common types are autosomal dominant and are characterized by hyperextensibility and fragility of the skin and hypermobility of the joints. There may be a bleeding tendency. The skin has a velvety feel and a fold may be easily stretched returning to its normal position when released. The skin tends to split as a result of relatively minor trauma. Joints are easily dislocated and the condition may present with congenital dislocation of the hip.

Erythropoietic protoporphyria (Figure 2.7) is an uncommon but not rare condition presenting as photosensitivity by the age of 2 years. Affected infants are fractious when placed in direct sunlight and older children dislike outdoor activities. Burning or tingling of the face and hands occurs after exposure to sunlight (ultraviolet wavelength is in the 400 nm and longer visible range) and serous crusts may form on the nose. The affected areas develop fine scars. There is an increased incidence of cholelithiasis. Transient fluorescence of red blood cells confirms the diagnosis. Oral beta-carotene/canthaxanthine (Roche) is a helpful protective agent in many affected individuals.

Ichthyosis

Ichthyosis vulgaris (Figures 2.8–2.11) which is often associated with atopic eczema, is the commonest of the many ichthyotic disorders. Excessive scaling usually appears during early childhood. The scales are generally small, white, and fine with the flexures characteristically spared. However, over the shins scales are often large, resembling fish-scales. Accentuated palmar markings are usual. Spontaneous improvement is common after puberty. Symptomatic treatment consists of hydration, use of emollient applications and many bath oils are also available.

Epidermolytic hyperkeratosis (bullous ichthyosiform erythroderma) (Figures 2.12, 2.13)
In this condition areas of epidermis peel off shortly after birth leaving raw areas and the appearance may suggest epidermolysis bullosa. The next stage is of crops of bullae which burst to leave raw areas that heal rapidly. The background skin is erythematous. In time warty hyperkeratosis becomes more prominent, appearing linear in the flexures. Histopathology reveals hydropic degeneration of the Malpighian cells. As the cells migrate up from the basal layer there is nuclear shrinkage and increasing vacuolation of the cytoplasm.

Neurofibromatosis (Figure 2.14)
Multiple benign tumours of neural tissue and multiple café-au-lait patches are usual. Although the café-au-lait patches may be present at birth, the neurofibromas do not develop until late childhood. Bilateral axillary freckling is pathognomonic of neuro-fibromatosis. Soft tumours can give the impression of being pushed through a button-hole defect in the skin. Congenital bone anomalies are not uncommon and tumours of brain, spinal cord and peripheral nerves occur.

Peutz–Jeghers syndrome (Figure 2.15) consists of the association of mucocutaneous lentigines with polyposis of the small and/or large intestine. The pigmented macules,

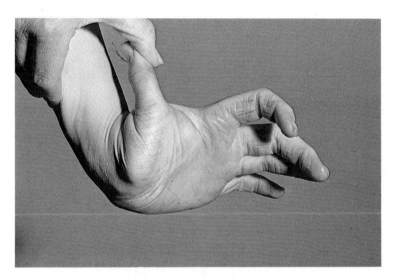

Figure 2.5   **Ehlers–Danlos syndrome** showing joint hypermobility.

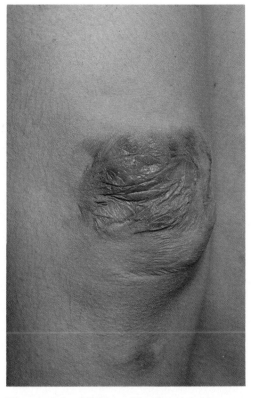

Figure 2.6   **Ehlers–Danlos syndrome** Characteristic thin scars with wrinkling of the skin, but also some fibrosis following haematoma resolution.

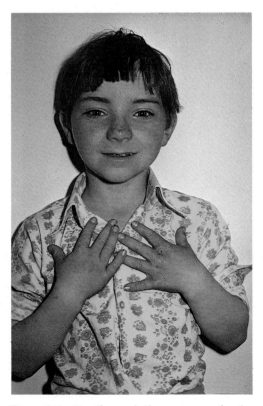

Figure 2.7   **Erythropoietic protoporphyria** Lesions over nose and knuckles which leave characteristic scars.

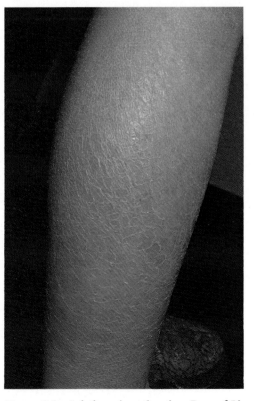

Figure 2.8   **Ichthyosis vulgaris**   Boy of $5\frac{1}{2}$ years.

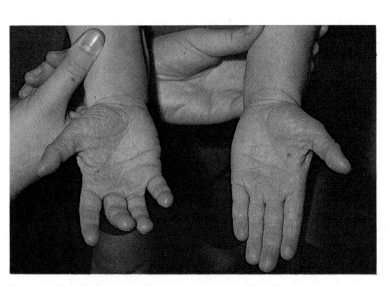

Figure 2.9 **Ichthyosis vulgaris** Same boy showing increased palmar markings.

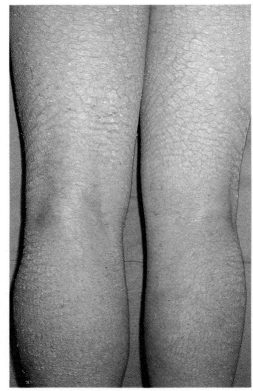

Figure 2.10 **Ichthyosis vulgaris** showing typical sparing of popliteal fossae.

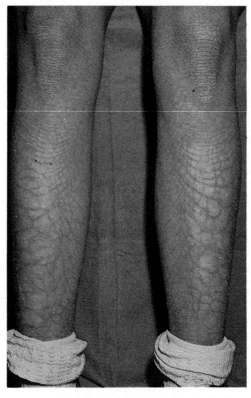

Figure 2.11 **Ichthyosis vulgaris** Girl of 13 with much larger scales over legs.

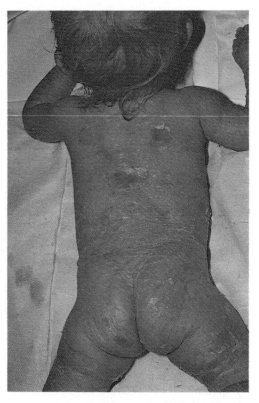

Figure 2.12 **Epidermolytic hyperkeratosis** One-year-old girl with reddened eroded skin since birth. (Courtesy of Dr M. Molokhia)

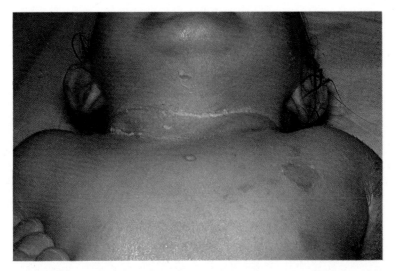

Figure 2.13 **Epidermolytic hyperkeratosis** Same child showing neck involvement and burst blisters. (Courtesy of Dr M. Molokhia)

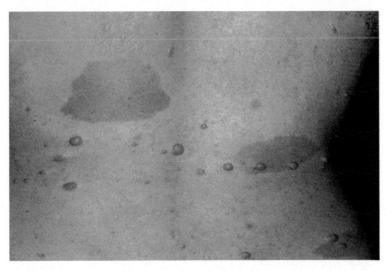

Figure 2.14 **Neurofibromatosis** Café-au-lait patches and tumours are visible.

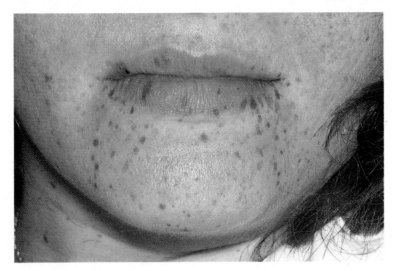

Figure 2.15 **Peutz–Jeghers syndrome** Multiple small lentigines over lips and adjacent skin.

unlike freckles, do show an increase in the number of melanocytes in the basal epidermal layer. Although the intestinal polyps are usually benign there is a slight but definite increased risk of gastrointestinal carcinoma. Small bowel polyps may bleed, leading to anaemia, and they also cause intussusception.

Tuberous sclerosis (Figures 2.16–2.18) is primarily a defect of connective tissue. The skin lesions often termed adenoma sebaceum but actually angiofibromata, usually appear towards the end of the first decade as small red-brown papules on the nose and naso-labial folds. They are often mistaken for acne, which can be distinguished by its more peripheral distribution, the presence of blackheads, and its tendency to form pustules. Other characteristic lesions are fibromas of the nail folds, irregularly coarsened skin over the sacrum (shagreen patch), and oval hypopigmented areas (ash leaf macules) which are often present in the neonate.

Tylosis (diffuse palmoplantar keratoderma) (Figure 2.19) is the commonest form of inherited localized thickening of skin over palms and soles. It manifests in early infancy as diffuse but well-defined smooth hyperkeratosis of palms and soles. Fissuring may be a problem in severe cases. A rare association between tylosis appearing in childhood rather than infancy, oral preleukoplakia and/or leukoplakia in tylotic children and adults, and the development of oesophageal carcinoma in adult life has been described in two Liverpool families.

AUTOSOMAL RECESSIVE

The parents of an affected individual commonly show no signs of the condition, but one in four of the progeny of heterozygote parents will be affected. Consanguinity is an important marker of recessive inheritance.

Acrodermatitis enteropathica (Figures 2.20–2.22) is seen particularly in infants at the time of weaning. Exudative eczematous lesions appear around the orifices and over scalp, hands and feet, and there is hair loss from the scalp, eyebrows and eyelashes. Diarrhoea is also present. The inherited condition is thought to be due to a defect in the absorption of zinc from the bowel. Oral zinc sulphate effectively reverses the condition. An acquired zinc-deficiency syndrome may also be seen in premature infants whether breast-fed or receiving total parenteral nutrition.

Ichthyosis

Non-bullous ichthyosiform erythroderma (Figure 2.23) may present as a 'collodion baby' in which case the true nature will become apparent after the membrane peels off. However, it can also present as such at birth, in which case the entire skin is dull red but particularly in the flexures. Superimposed on the erythema is hyperkeratosis so that the skin looks and feels thicker and more rigid than normal. The rigidity of the skin may result in ectropion. The severity of the condition varies but most patients survive, showing generalized faint erythema and hyperkeratosis, most marked over palms and soles, as time goes on.

Lamellar ichthyosis (Figures 2.24, 2.25) can be considered a form of non-bullous ichthy-osiform erythroderma in which large greyish-brown scales with raised edges occur.

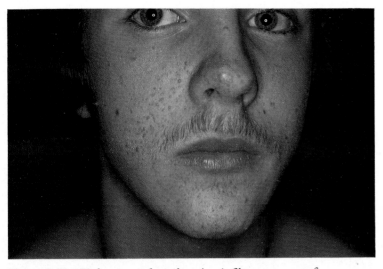

Figure 2.16 **Tuberous sclerosis** Angiofibromata over face.

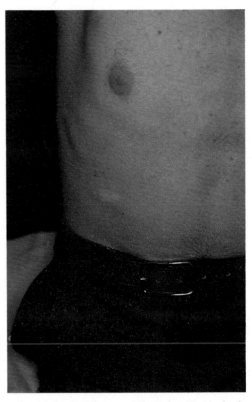

Figure 2.17 **Tuberous sclerosis** Typical ash leaf macule over right lower chest.

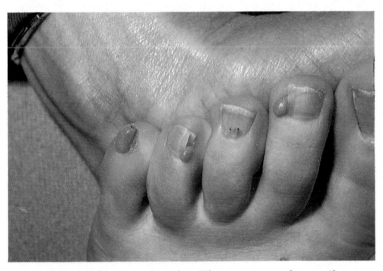

Figure 2.18 **Tuberous sclerosis** Fibromata around toe-nails.

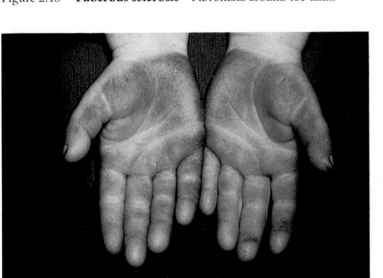

Figure 2.19 **Tylosis** The change from normal to affected skin is well-defined.

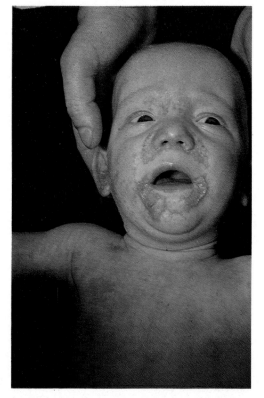

Figure 2.20 **Acrodermatitis enteropathica** Male of 4 months with typical moist perioral eruption.

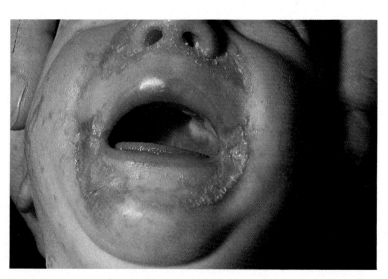

Figure 2.21 **Acrodermatitis enteropathica** Close-up of same infant.

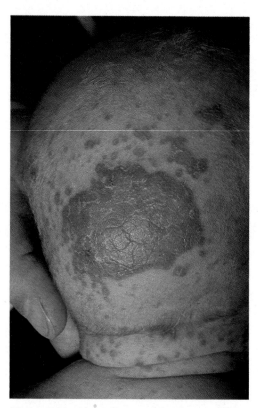

Figure 2.22 **Acrodermatitis enteropathica** Same infant with fiery eczematous-looking patches over head. No *Candida* was grown from any site.

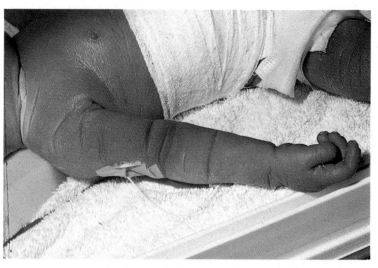

Figure 2.23 **Non-bullous ichthyosiform erythroderma** Two-day-old baby showing raised, thickened erythematous skin.

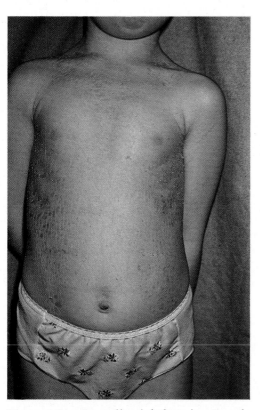

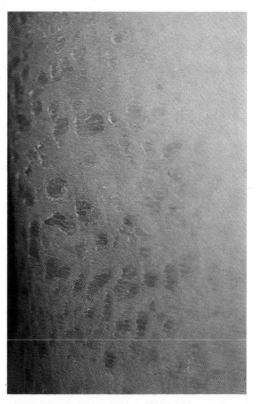

Figure 2.24 **Lamellar ichthyosis** Female of nearly 5 years with involvement of neck and sides of trunk. Midline back was more mildly affected and she had large scales over scalp. She was a collodion baby. (Figures 3.8–3.11 show her as a baby)

Figure 2.25 **Lamellar ichthyosis** Close-up of right-side chest of same child showing plate-like scales with elevated edges.

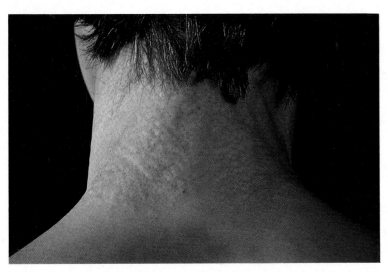

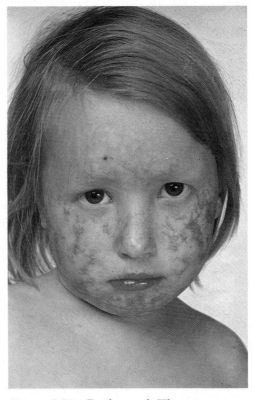

Figure 2.26 **Pseudoxanthoma elasticum** Plucked-chicken skin appearance over back of neck.

Figure 2.27 **Rothmund–Thomson syndrome** Widespread facial telangiectasia is shown.

Pseudoxanthoma elasticum (Figure 2.26)

There are two autosomal dominant forms and two autosomal recessive forms of this generalized disorder of elastin, but most cases are recessive. The condition does not usually manifest until the second decade of life or later. The skin, eyes and cardiovascular system are affected. The skin lesions are yellow oval papules that arise particularly on neck, in the axillae, cubital fossae, and inguinal and periumbilical areas. The appearance of lesions is pebbly and has been likened to a crepe bandage or plucked chicken skin.

Rothmund–Thomson syndrome (poikiloderma congenitale) (Figures 2.27, 2.28) is rare and characterized by atrophy, pigmentation and telangiectasia of the skin in association with juvenile cataracts, short stature, partial or total alopecia, defects of nails and teeth and hypogonadism. It is more common in females. Skin changes generally appear in the first six months of life. There is light sensitivity with erythema with or without blisters occurring on exposed skin, although the subsequent poikiloderma and other changes are not in fact confined to sites of exposure.

Xeroderma pigmentosum (Figures 2.29, 2.30) is a rare condition characterized by hypersensitivity to ultraviolet rays followed eventually by the development of multiple solar keratoses, cutaneous basal and squamous cell carcinomas and malignant melanomas in exposed areas. Photosensitivity may be apparent from the age of 2 months, erythema occurring over exposed areas, particularly the face. After a few years of exposure the skin becomes dry, with freckles, hypopigmentation, atrophy and scarring. Patients usually die in childhood from metastasis of the tumours. The cause is a defect of the normal repair mechanism of DNA damaged by ultraviolet rays. The condition can now be identified before birth.

X-LINKED DOMINANT

A heterozygote female transmits the disease to 50% of her sons and transmits the carrier state to 50% of her daughters. Males and heterozygous females manifest the condition.

Focal dermal hypoplasia (Goltz syndrome) (Figures 2.31, 2.32) manifests as scar-like lesions, atrophy and telangiectasia, and over the face the appearance may simulate overuse of topical corticosteroids. Hypotrichosis, and short, partially absent brittle nails are common. Subcutaneous fat covered only by epidermis may occur over posterior thigh, groin, and iliac crest areas. The trait is often prenatally lethal in the male.

Incontinentia pigmenti (Bloch–Sulzberger syndrome) (Figure 2.33) usually presents within a few days of birth and is usually prenatally lethal in males, the few surviving males being the result of spontaneous mutation. Linear or grouped vesicles appear on the trunk and limbs but by the end of the first month blistering disappears and is followed by the appearance of small firm papules and warty plaques. The papules in turn involute leaving angulated and streaked pigmentation. The condition is frequently associated with dental, skeletal, eye and central nervous system abnormalities.

X-LINKED RECESSIVE

A heterozygote female transmits the condition to 50% of her sons and transmits the carrier state to 50% of her daughters. Heterozygous females may show some signs of the condition.

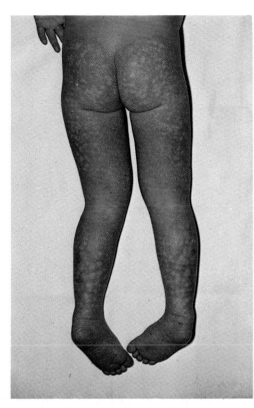

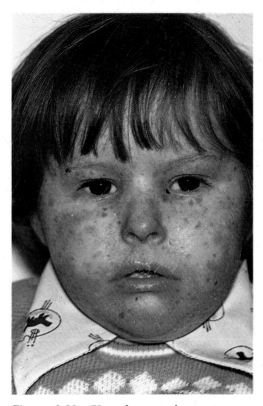

Figure 2.28 **Rothmund–Thomson syndrome** Poikilodermatous change over buttocks and lower limbs is visible.

Figure 2.29 **Xeroderma pigmentosum** This child already shows atrophy, tightness, hypopigmentation and dryness of the skin.

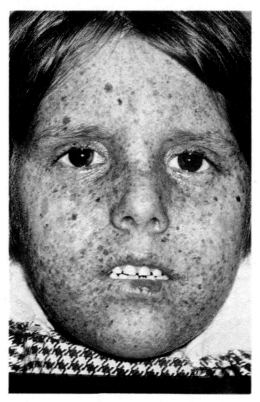

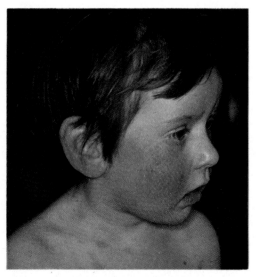

Figure 2.30 **Xeroderma pigmentosum** Another child demonstrating a later stage with multiple pigmented lesions, solar keratoses, and lip ulceration.

Figure 2.31 **Focal dermal hypoplasia** showing erythema of cheek with depressed scar-like lesions here. This child also had patches of aplasia cutis over the scalp.

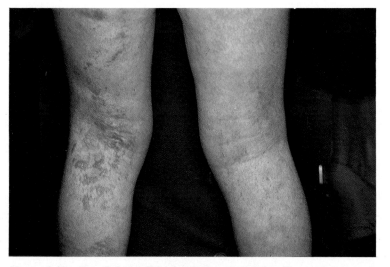

Figure 2.32 **Focal dermal hypoplasia** Reddish-yellow subcutaneous fat covered only by epidermis is visible over the left popliteal fossa.

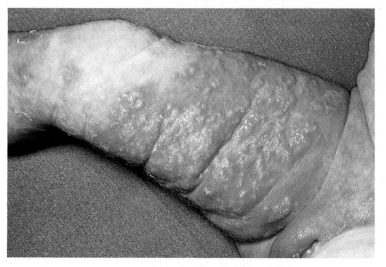

Figure 2.33 **Incontinentia pigmenti** Blisters over a lower limb.

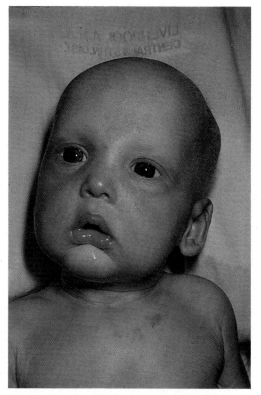

Figure 2.34 **Anhidrotic ectodermal dysplasia** Two-month-old baby showing typical facies with wrinkled periorbital skin, absent eyebrows and eyelashes, small chin and pouting lower lip.

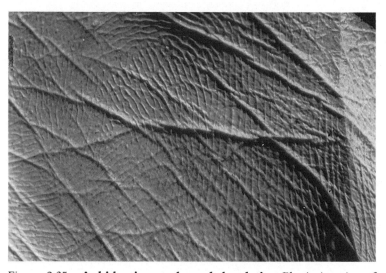

Figure 2.35 **Anhidrotic ectodermal dysplasia** Plastic imprint of left hypothenar area, same infant at same age, showing flattened ridges and absent pores (× 14).

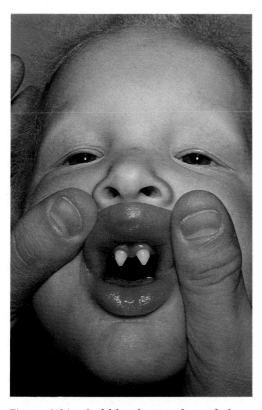

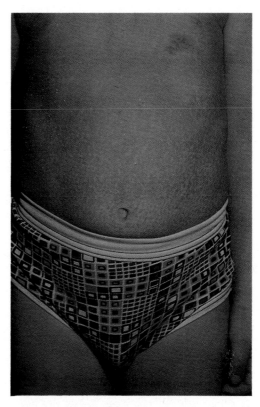

Figure 2.36 **Anhidrotic ectodermal dysplasia** Another child aged 3 years showing characteristic pointed 'tiger teeth'.

Figure 2.37 **Sex-linked ichthyosis** Boy of 3½ years. Note the dark scales. The front of the trunk was more severely affected than the back. He has a coincidental resolving haemangioma inferior to the left breast.

Ectodermal dysplasia

Anhidrotic ectodermal dysplasia (Figures 2.34–2.36) patients tend to show a similar facial appearance with the nose saddle-shaped with a depressed bridge, the chin small and pointed and the forehead bossed. The skin tends to be pale, soft, thin, dry and shiny. Periorbital skin is wrinkled and hyperpigmented. Scalp hair is short, fine and scanty, and eyebrows and eyelashes sparse or absent. Atopic eczema may be present. There is abnormal, delayed or absent dentition, affecting both the deciduous and permanent teeth. The deciduous teeth are widely spaced and conical. Eccrine sweat glands are absent or diminished in number and total sweating is slight. It should be noted that in the infant, the characteristic features of the condition are often inapparent and fever of obscure origin may be the only manifestation. It must be emphasized that an infective cause should always be looked for in febrile episodes and treated accordingly.

Ichthyosis

X-linked ichthyosis (Figure 2.37) is less common but more severe than ichthyosis vulgaris. The scales tend to be much larger, polygonal, and have a dirty-brown or black colour. The scaliness is frequently obvious at birth. The entire skin surface, including flexures and scalp, may be affected but if the face is involved it is usually only the sides, and increased palm and sole markings are not a feature. The condition is persistent. Steroid sulphatase deficiency is associated with this disorder and its absence permits identification of maternal carriers.

3

The newborn

TOXIC ERYTHEMA OF THE NEWBORN (Figure 3.1) begins within 48 hours of birth and disappears in a few days. Blotchy erythematous macules 2–3 cm in diameter with a central vesicle appear over trunk, face or limbs. Smear of the vesicle reveals numerous eosinophils. This common benign condition is of unknown cause.

CUTIS MARMORATA (Figure 3.2) is a normal reticulated bluish mottling of the skin seen on the trunk and extremities of infants and young children. It is a physiological response to chilling with resultant dilatation of capillaries and small venules and (unlike livedo reticularis) disappears as the infant is rewarmed.

MILIA (Figure 3.3) commonly occur on the face of the newborn and result from retention of keratin and sebaceous material within the pilosebaceous apparatus of the neonate. They appear as multiple pearly-white or yellow 1–2 mm papules. These keratin cysts usually rupture on to the skin surface and disappear within a few weeks of birth.

SEBACEOUS GLAND HYPERPLASIA (Figures 3.4, 3.5) is manifested by multiple yellow tiny papules on nose, cheeks and upper lips of newborn infants. They are a manifestation of maternal androgen stimulation and are a temporary phenomenon resolving in a few weeks. Although sometimes considered the same as milia, the sebaceous hyperplasia papules tend to be more florid and are not cystic.

MILIARIA (Figures 3.6, 3.7) caused by eccrine sweat retention is characterized by an erythematous papulo-vesicular eruption that is distributed particularly over face, neck, upper chest and back, but wherever there is excessive heating of the skin. Therapy is directed towards avoidance of excessive heat and humidity, with lightweight loose clothing recommended.

COLLODION BABY (Figures 3.8–3.12) describes an appearance rather than a specific disease. These babies are born enveloped in a shiny transparent but fairly rigid membrane which cracks and peels off after a few days, and at this time the true skin appearance of the child can be visualized. In fact, many of these children will have no

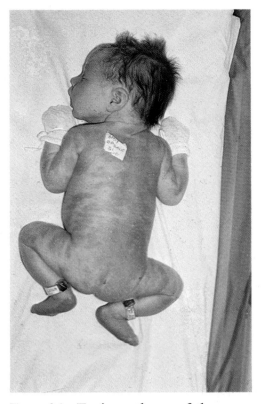

Figure 3.1 **Toxic erythema of the newborn** The typical blotchy patches, each with a central vesicle are visible.

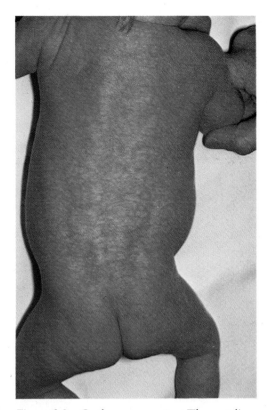

Figure 3.2 **Cutis marmorata** The mottling disappeared on rewarming the skin.

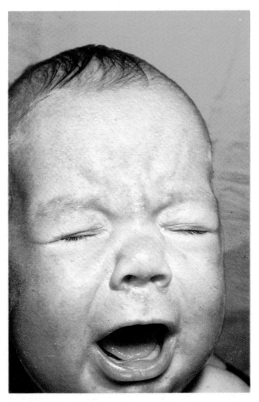

Figure 3.3 **Milia** The small white papules can be seen over the forehead.

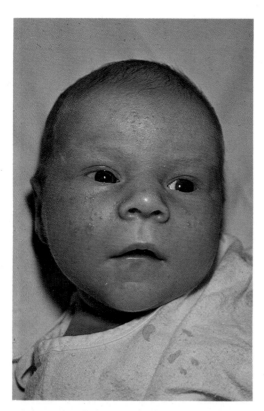

Figure 3.4 **Sebaceous gland hyperplasia**
23-day-old infant showing florid yellow
papules.

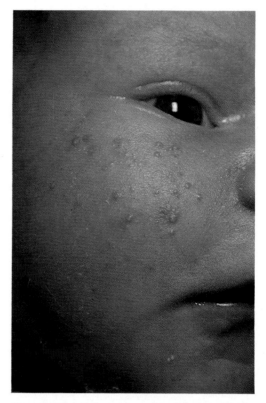

Figure 3.5 **Sebaceous gland hyperplasia**
Close-up of same child.

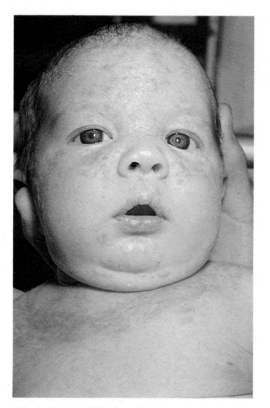

Figure 3.6 **Miliaria** Vesicles are clearly visible on an erythematous background.

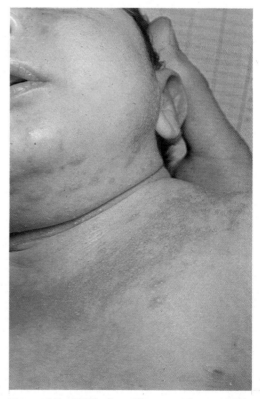

Figure 3.7 **Miliaria** Close-up of same child.

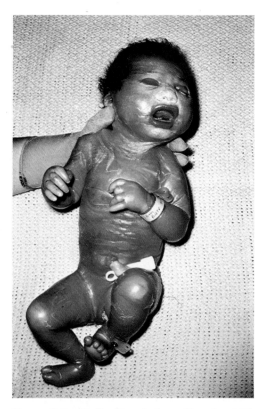

Figure 3.8 **Collodion baby** Female child on first day of life.

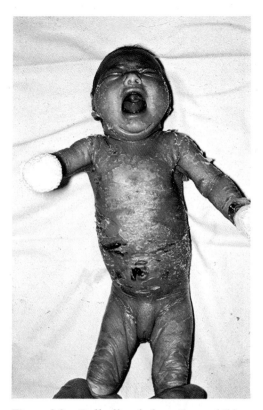

Figure 3.9 **Collodion baby** Same child at 6 days.

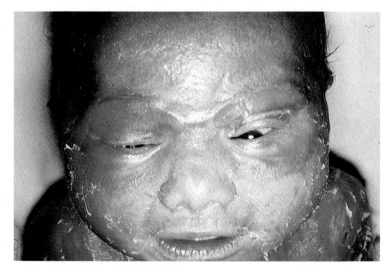

Figure 3.10 **Collodion baby** Close-up of face at 6 days.

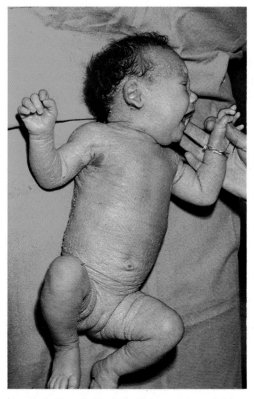

Figure 3.11 **Collodion baby** Same child at 27 days showing how membrane has separated, revealing dry skin. The same child is pictured nearly 5 years later with mild lamellar ichthyosis in Chapter 2, Figures 2.24, 2.25.

underlying disorder but an appreciable number will have non-bullous ichthyosiform erythroderma, lamellar ichthyosis, X-linked ichthyosis, or ichthyosis vulgaris.

NAPKIN AREA ERUPTIONS

Napkin (irritant, diaper) dermatitis (Figures 3.13–3.20) is an irritant frictional contact dermatitis and the most common eruption in the napkin area. It is unusual in the first month of life. It may occur alone or with other napkin-area eruptions. Contact with napkin material soaked in urine irritates the skin of susceptible infants and urea-splitting organisms in faeces or infected urine increase the alkalinity and the likelihood of a dermatitis. Thus, diarrhoea or soiled napkins left on for prolonged periods encourage the appearance of dermatitis. However, this condition is not synonymous with ammoniacal dermatitis although this term can be correctly applied to some eroded forms.

Disinfectant, soap, soap powder, detergent or talc persisting in inadequately rinsed napkins produce frictional damage to the skin and too vigorous cleansing of the nappy area can be traumatic. Some nappy liners increase frictional irritation and may cause a W-shaped dermatitis; pure terylene liners are safer. Clinically, napkin dermatitis appears as a patchy or diffuse erythema in the napkin area, as discrete erosions, ulcers, or herpetiform lesions which dry or burst. The eruption favours convexities. Untreated, the inflamed skin can sometimes extend over the back and down the inner thighs and simulate scalding. Secondary bacterial and candidal infection is common and either staphylococcal or sterile pustules due to sweat retention (miliaria) are often present.

Infantile gluteal granuloma (Figure 3.21) is the term describing large erythematous nodules appearing on a background of napkin dermatitis. They resolve spontaneously, but often months after the original napkin dermatitis has resolved.

Infantile seborrhoeic dermatitis (Figures 3.22–3.27) is a non-irritant condition that typically occurs within the first three months of life but usually in the first few weeks, and clears within weeks of its onset. Relevant to its cause may be the fact that, under the influence of maternal androgen, there is sebaceous gland activity in the first few months of life. Although the condition is distinct from atopic dermatitis there does appear to be an increased incidence of atopic dermatitis appearing later in these children. The relationship, if any, between this condition and seborrhoeic dermatitis in adolescents or adults is unclear. The napkin area and particularly the groins, or the scalp, are the common sites of onset but axillae, neck, and post-auricular regions are also usually affected. Erythema, maceration, and scaling involve the skin folds and the adjacent area, but frequently erythema and discrete lesions with greasy-looking scales become more widespread over the trunk and face. Although yellowish greasy scaling of the scalp may be the only manifestation in some infants, very occasionally infantile seborrhoeic dermatitis can become a generalized erythroderma requiring hospitalization. Local candidal and bacterial infections often complicate infantile seborrhoeic dermatitis and oral thrush may also be present. Plastic pants worn over napkins increase the likelihood of infection occurring.

Napkin psoriasis (Figure 3.28) describes a napkin rash with a well-defined edge followed by a more widespread psoriasiform eruption, appearing in an infant of 8 months or younger. The reddish scaly plaques are not irritant and the condition is self-limiting,

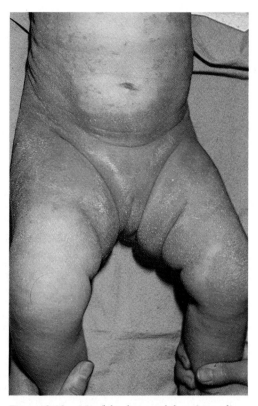

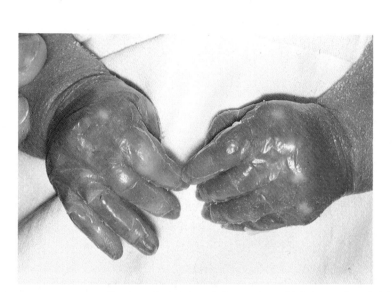

Figure 3.12 **Collodion baby** Another 1-day-old baby. This child had normal skin when the membrane separated.

Figure 3.13 **Napkin dermatitis** Spreading scald appearance over napkin area. *Staphylococcus aureus* complicated the eruption.

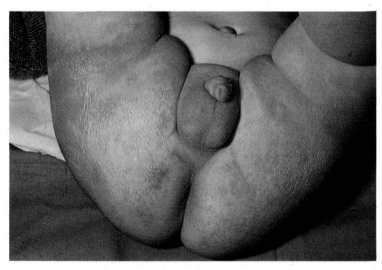

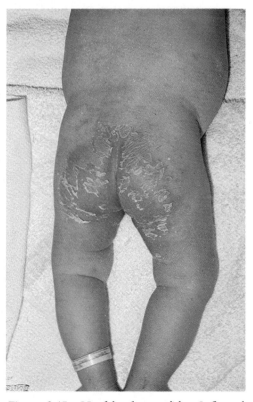

Figure 3.14 **Napkin dermatitis** Scald type with well-defined edges and convexities affected.

Figure 3.15 **Napkin dermatitis** Inflamed and peeling skin over buttocks and inner thighs.

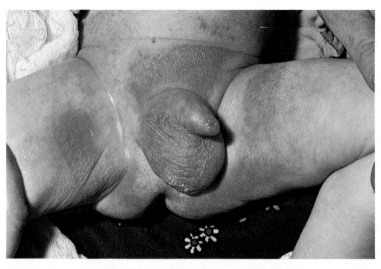

Figure 3.16 **Napkin dermatitis** W-shaped dermatitis sparing the groins.

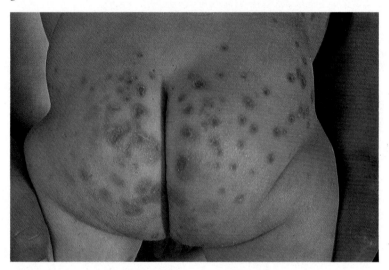

Figure 3.17 **Napkin dermatitis** Superficial erosive type.

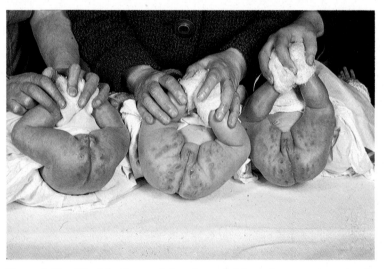

Figure 3.18 **Napkin dermatitis** Superficial erosive type occurring in triplets.

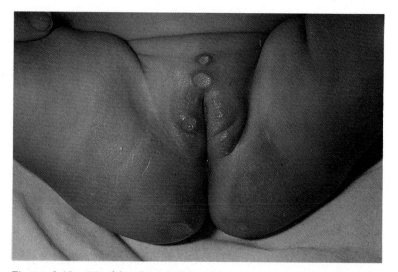

Figure 3.19 **Napkin dermatitis** More severe erosive type. This infant has an ammoniacal dermatitis.

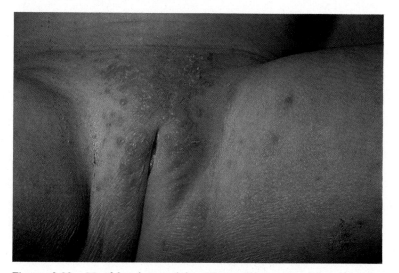

Figure 3.20 **Napkin dermatitis** Herpetiform type. These vesicles rapidly dried up. No organism grew on culture.

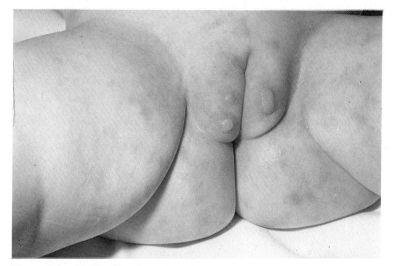

Figure 3.21 **Infantile gluteal granuloma** Typical soft nodules involving the vulva in this infant.

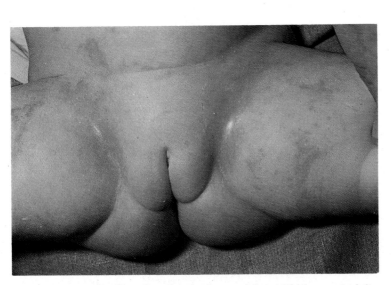

Figure 3.22 **Infantile seborrhoeic dermatitis** Mild but typical distribution which began at age of 2 weeks.

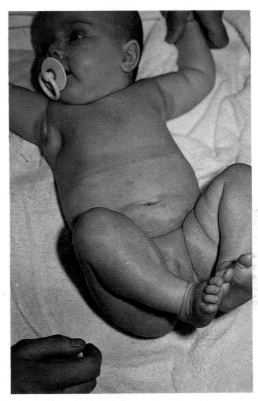

Figure 3.23 **Infantile seborrhoeic dermatitis** showing involvement of the napkin area and axillae.

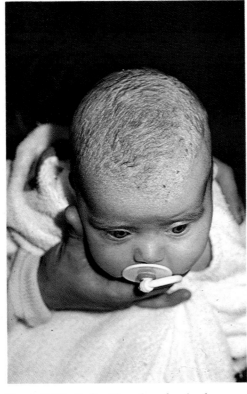

Figure 3.24 **Infantile seborrhoeic dermatitis** Same baby showing scalp involvement.

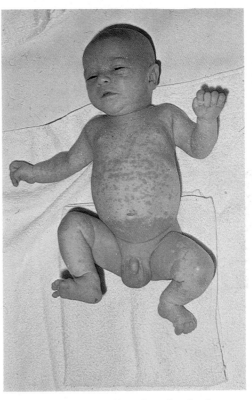

Figure 3.25 **Infantile seborrhoeic dermatitis** Widespread eruption.

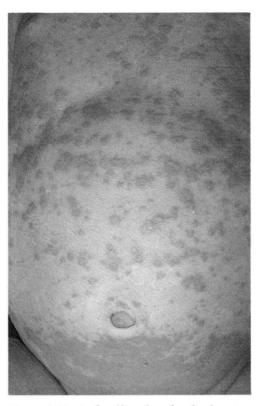

Figure 3.26 **Infantile seborrhoeic derma-titis** Close-up of trunk of same baby.

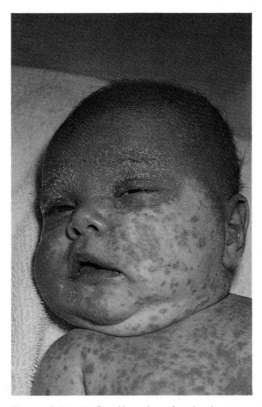

Figure 3.27 **Infantile seborrhoeic derma-titis** Severe facial involvement in a 1-month-old baby.

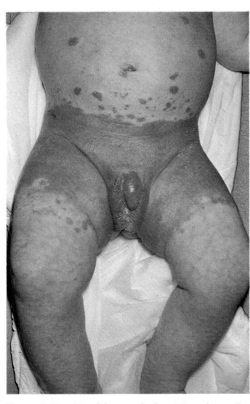

Figure 3.28 **Napkin psoriasis** Note the well-defined napkin area eruption with psoriasiform spread.

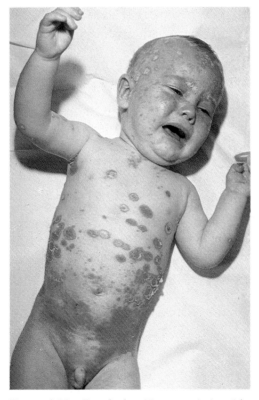

Figure 3.29 **Psoriasis** True psoriasis with onset at 7 weeks of age.

lasting a few weeks. Candidal infection is sometimes a complicating factor. It seems likely that the napkin psoriasis is really infantile seborrhoeic dermatitis in a psoriasis-prone individual.

Psoriasis (Figures 3.29, 3.30) is rare before the age of 2 years but we have seen an occasional infant of a few months old who clearly had true psoriasis. Follow-up of such children over a period of years indicates that lesions tend to be persistent and remissions are few and far between.

Candidiasis (Figure 3.31) presents as a moist erythematous eruption often with satellite pustules, predominantly over the buttocks and perianal region. Oral antibiotic therapy predisposes to the condition which can be treated with nystatin or miconazole cream. Oral candidiasis will also require treatment.

Scabies (Figures 3.32, 3.33) must not be forgotten in the itching newborn infant and if the napkin area is involved papules will be visible and evidence of scabies over palms, soles, and trunk will be found. Other members of the family should be examined and treated in addition to the baby. For the baby, after initial bathing and change of bedding we use half-strength benzyl benzoate application BP applied twice to the entire skin below the neck and then once again the following morning. For any definite burrows above the neck crotamiton ointment can be used. Gamma benzene hexachloride in a 1% cream or lotion is an alternative treatment for scabies and we recommend a single application below the neck left on for 8–12 hours only.

Perianal dermatitis (Figure 3.34)
A localized perianal dermatitis is common after an attack of diarrhoea but may also form part of an irritant dermatitis or infantile seborrhoeic dermatitis.

INTERTRIGO (Figure 3.35) is a moist erythematous eruption where there is friction between opposed skin surfaces. It is seen particularly in overweight infants; groins, neck and axillae are common sites. The eruption is usually localized to the frictional site unlike infantile seborrhoea which extends beyond these areas.

STAPHYLOCOCCAL INFECTIONS
Staphylococcal scalded skin syndrome (Figures 3.36–3.38) may be preceded by a purulent conjunctivitis, otitis media, or an upper respiratory infection. Staphylococci can be isolated from such foci. A widespread tender erythema then develops within a few hours to a few days, and is worse over face, neck, axillae and groins. This is followed by the appearance of large flaccid bullae. The upper portion of the epidermis peels away exposing raw scald-like areas. Mucosae can be affected. Sometimes the eruption may be more localized, and widespread erythema without blistering is also seen. Pustules are rare in this condition except in the napkin and periumbilical areas of neonates. Recovery without scarring is usually within 5–7 days with or without administration of antibiotics. We feel it safer to treat all cases with penicillinase-resistant penicillin or fusidic acid. The rash is due to production of an exotoxin from phage group 2 benzyl penicillin-resistant staphylococci. There is often a history of typical impetigo in a sibling.

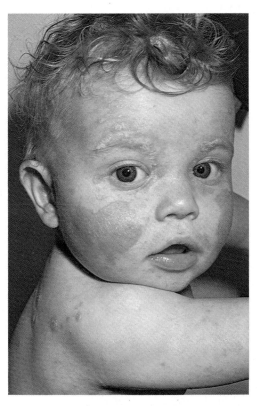

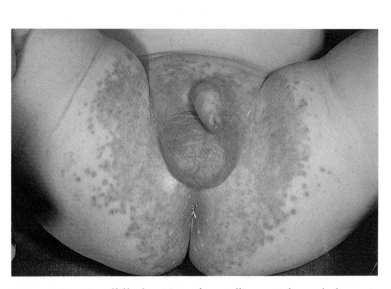

Figure 3.30 **Psoriasis** True psoriasis with onset before 2 months old. This child, now aged 9 years, has had persistent psoriasis, poorly responsive to topical treatment.

Figure 3.31 **Candidiasis** Note the satellite pustules and the main eruption.

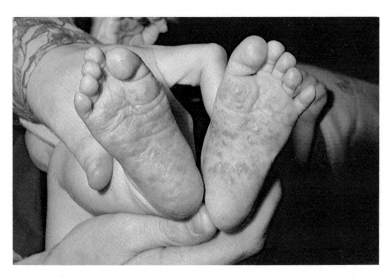

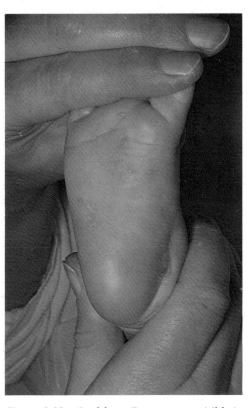

Figure 3.32 **Scabies** In infants, papules, pustules and vesicles affecting soles are common.

Figure 3.33 **Scabies** Burrows are visible in this 2-month-old baby.

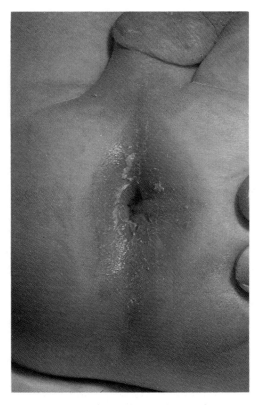

Figure 3.34   Perianal dermatitis   There was skin sepsis elsewhere in this baby.

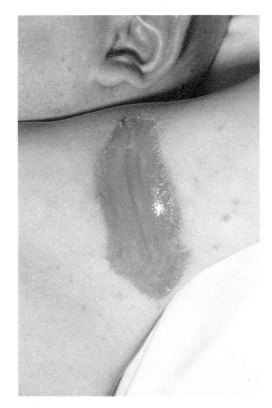

Figure 3.35   Intertrigo   This just involved the axillae in this overweight child.

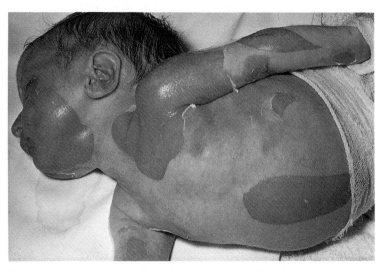

Figure 3.36   Staphylococcal scalded skin syndrome   The disorder was fatal in this severely affected child who died within the first week of life. Previously the term pemphigus neonatorum would have been used.

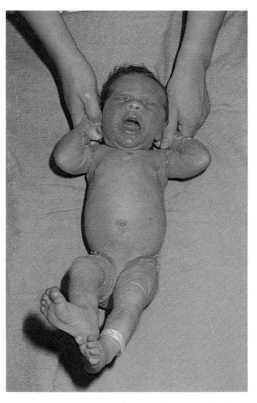

Figure 3.37   Staphylococcal scalded skin syndrome   Another baby aged 2 weeks with lesions showing a tendency to localization.

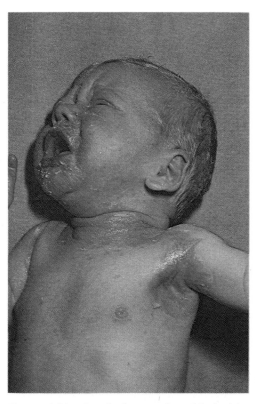

Figure 3.38 **Staphylococcal scalded skin syndrome** Close-up of a similarly affected 12-day-old child showing facial erythema and perioral, neck and axillary involvement.

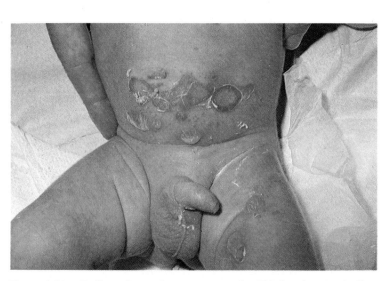

Figure 3.39 **Bullous impetigo** Two-week-old baby showing bullae, some of which clearly show a fluid level of pus. Began at 9 days.

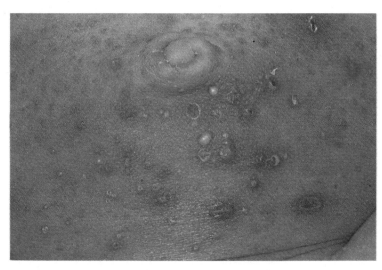

Figure 3.40 **Bullous impetigo** This neonate seen at 13 days with vesicular rather than bullous lesions. Eruption was said to have started at 4 days. Benzyl penicillin-resistant *Staphylococcus aureus* grew on culture of pus.

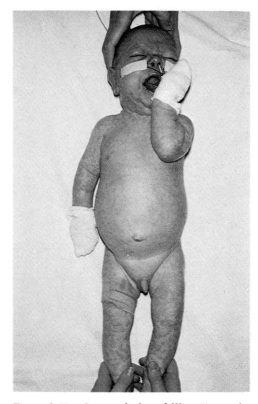

Figure 3.41 **Congenital syphilis** Six-week-old infant with hepatosplenomegaly and rash.

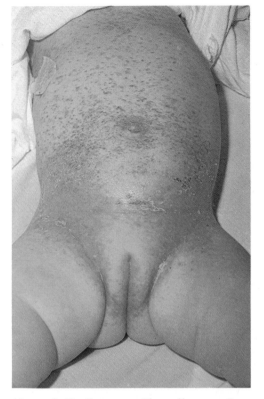

Figure 3.42 **Letterer–Siwe disease** Purpuric papular eruption over trunk. (There is also a true infantile seborrhoeic dermatitis involving the napkin area)

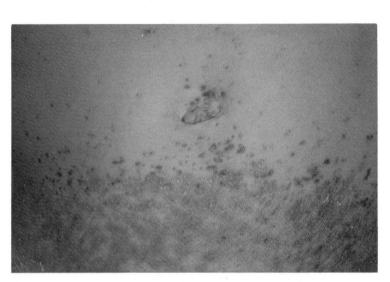

Figure 3.43 **Letterer–Siwe disease** Close-up of purpuric papular eruption involving lower trunk in another baby. (Courtesy of Dr T. W. Stewart)

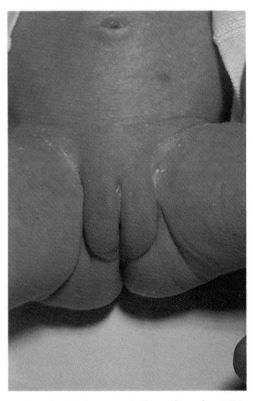

Figure 3.44 **Letterer–Siwe disease** This baby was noticed to have a vesico-pustule on a heel at birth and then developed a few other sterile pustules in the following week. Two lesions are visible over vulva and abdomen.

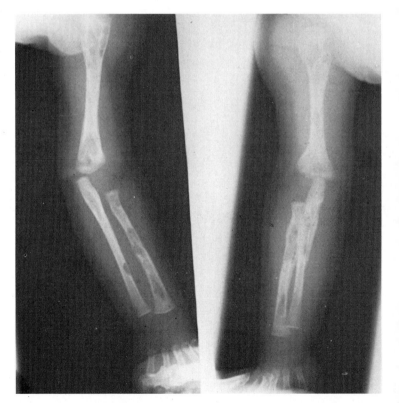

Figure 3.45 **Letterer–Siwe disease** Same child 6–7 weeks later. The infant cried with pain when lifted and was found to have multiple skeletal lesions and consequent fractures. The child remains well following chemotherapy at that time, 6 years ago.

Bullous impetigo (Figures 3.39, 3.40)

A purely bullous or vesicular form of impetigo is seen particularly in the newborn, lesions of which only grow staphylococci on culture. It may be that bullous impetigo is a localized form of staphyloccoccal scalded skin syndrome.

CONGENITAL SYPHILIS (Figure 3.41) is a disorder in which the fetus becomes infected with organisms by way of the placenta, usually sometime after the 16th week of pregnancy. Infants with congenital syphilis often show no external signs of disease at the time of birth. The common clinical manifestations in early congenital syphilis include anaemia, fever, hepatosplenomegaly, lymphadenopathy, rhinitis, and mucocutaneous eruptions. Cutaneous eruptions are varied in character but discrete copper-brown maculo-papular or papulo-squamous lesions are most common.

LETTERER–SIWE DISEASE (Figures 3.42–3.45) is a form of histiocytosis X which usually presents with an infantile seborrhoeic dermatitis-like distribution and appearance but uncommonly before the age of 9 months. On closer inspection, reddish-brown or purpuric papules may identify the disorder. In another form in infants vesicopustules may predominate. An affected infant with skin lesions may appear healthy for months before fever, anaemia, thrombocytopenia, adenopathy, hepatosplenomegaly, or skeletal tumours become apparent.

4
Atopic and other dermatitis

ATOPIC DERMATITIS (atopic eczema) (Figures 4.1–4.28)

The term atopy indicates an inherited tendency to develop one or more of a related group of common conditions (asthma, eczema of atopic type, hay fever, acute urticaria of allergic type), subject to much environmental influence. Perhaps 10% of the population of the United Kingdom are atopic and 3% of these will have atopic dermatitis. Raised IgE levels are found in 80% of atopics. There is evidence to suggest that atopy is caused by or associated with a lymphocyte defect.

Atopic dermatitis usually presents in the infant between the age of 3 months and 2 years. The atopic child often has a characteristic pallor, particularly of the face. One should note that the ability to have a co-ordinated scratch does not occur before the age of 2 months. The initial site of involvement of atopic dermatitis is commonly face and scalp and there is then spread to the extensor aspect of limbs. Although buttocks may be affected in infants one sometimes sees widespread skin involvement with sparing of the napkin area. Within months of onset cubital and popliteal fossae, lower buttock folds, and frictional areas such as neck, wrists and ankles, become affected and eczema may sometimes be localized to these areas. The dorsal aspect of hands and feet are other common sites. Lichenification with accentuation of skin markings is a common finding. Rubbing and scratching encourage secondary bacterial infection, and painless lymphadenopathy is frequently found with inflamed skin. Eczema beginning after the age of 2 years tends to have a poorer prognosis than when it presents earlier. Prolonged extensor limb involvement is also a bad prognostic sign. Atopic eczema skin is commonly dry, and may be dry enough to constitute ichthyosis vulgaris. It is, in fact, common for atopic dermatitis and ichthyosis vulgaris to co-exist, and about 50% of those with autosomal dominant ichthyosis have evidence of atopy. Dry skin whether associated with atopy or not, is prone to frictional irritant dermatitis. As in ichthyosis vulgaris, an increase in the number of palm and sole markings may be present. Patchy roughness of the skin particularly over the backs of the upper arms and front of thighs due to horny plugging of follicles is termed *keratosis pilaris* and is common both in atopics and non-atopics. Children with atopic eczema may show an extra infraorbital skin crease (or creases) which may occur as an isolated sign or be a sign of previous eczematous inflammation at that site. Other patterns of atopic dermatitis include eyelid

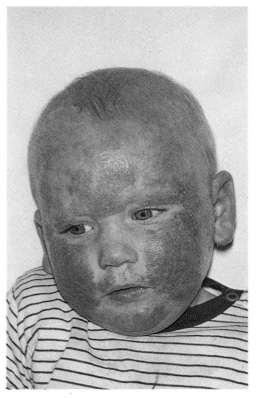

Figure 4.1 **Atopic dermatitis** Typical eczema over face in an infant.

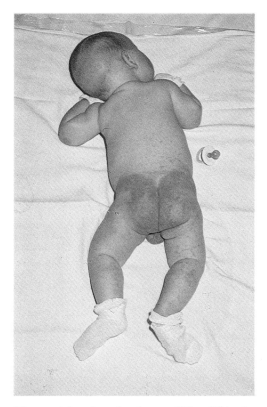

Figure 4.2 **Atopic dermatitis** This 5-month-old boy had typical facial dermatitis also.

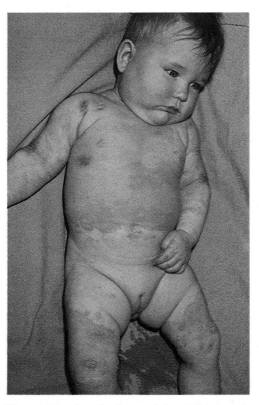

Figure 4.3 **Atopic dermatitis** Widespread eczema but sparing napkin area.

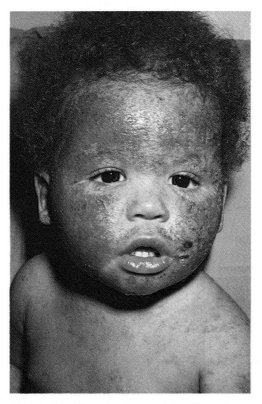

Figure 4.4 **Atopic dermatitis** Severe excoriated eczema in a 15-month-old child.

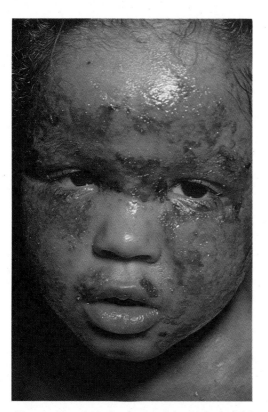

Figure 4.5 **Atopic dermatitis** Same child 3 years later with face worse and exudative.

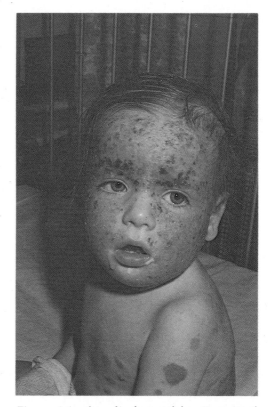

Figure 4.6 **Atopic dermatitis** Excoriated eczema.

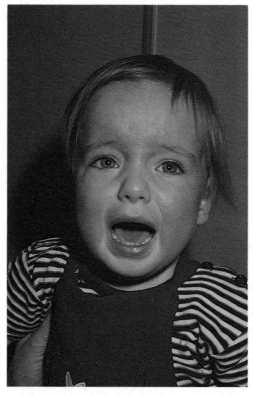

Figure 4.7 **Atopic dermatitis** Same child 9 days later with skin healed.

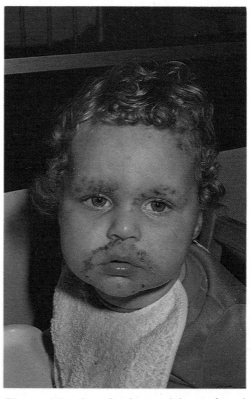

Figure 4.8 **Atopic dermatitis** Infected eczema face – more localized distribution.

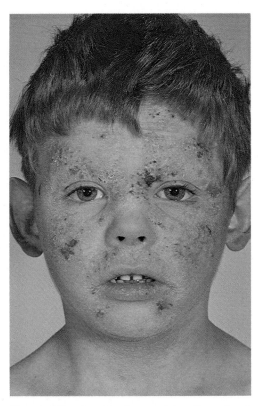

Figure 4.9 **Atopic dermatitis** Excoriated and infected eczema patches. Note the dry, pale skin.

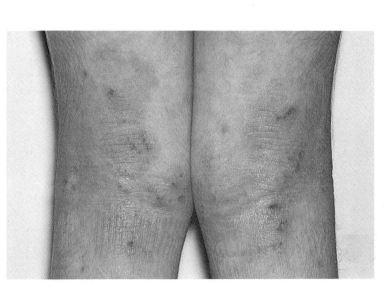

Figure 4.10 **Atopic dermatitis** Flexural involvement with lichenification.

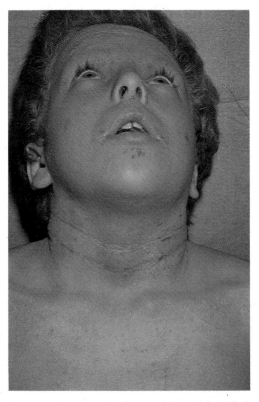

Figure 4.11 **Atopic dermatitis** Lichenified eczema affecting the neck in a boy of 10 – a common site.

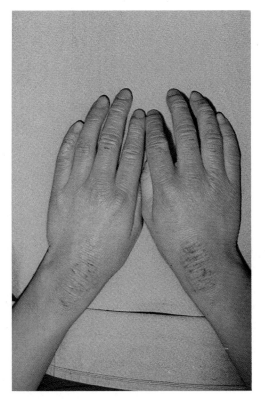

Figure 4.12 **Atopic dermatitis** Same boy with wrist involvement.

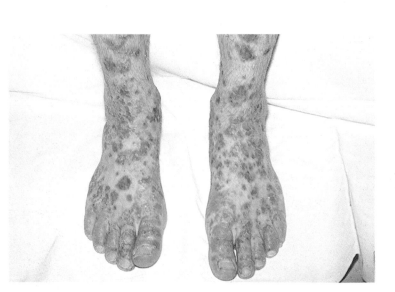

Figure 4.13   **Atopic dermatitis**   Excoriated eczema in an older child showing infected nummular lesions also.

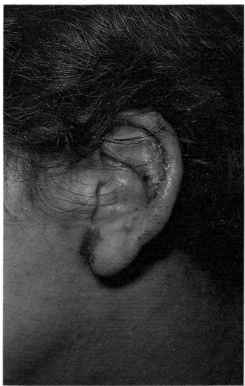

Figure 4.14   **Atopic dermatitis**   Same boy with infected ear eczema. Note involvement at junction of lobe with facial skin.

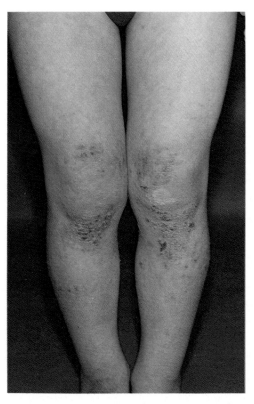

Figure 4.15   **Atopic dermatitis**   Boy of 4½ years with front of knees affected. He had only minimal flexor knee involvement.

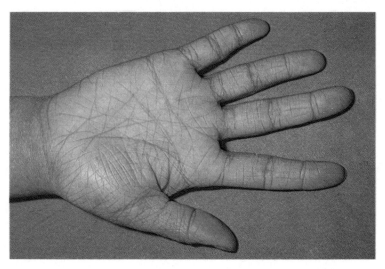

Figure 4.16   **Atopic dermatitis**   Increased palmar markings.

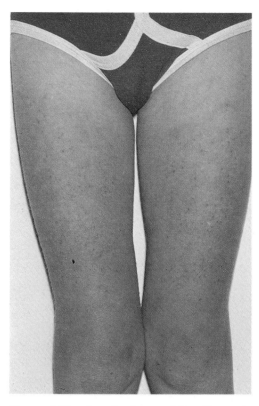

Figure 4.17 **Atopic dermatitis** Keratosis pilaris – thighs. Prominent follicles which have been rubbed, can be seen.

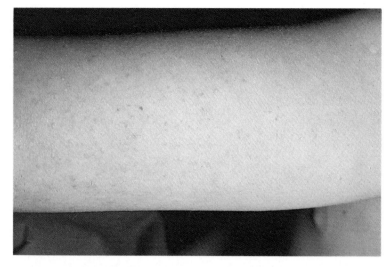

Figure 4.18 **Atopic dermatitis** Keratosis pilaris affecting the extensor aspect of upper arm.

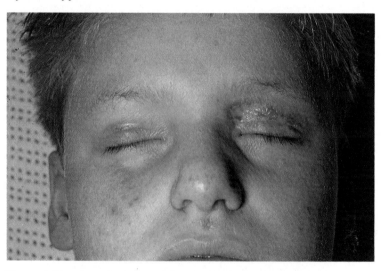

Figure 4.19 **Atopic dermatitis** Rubbed excoriated eyelids.

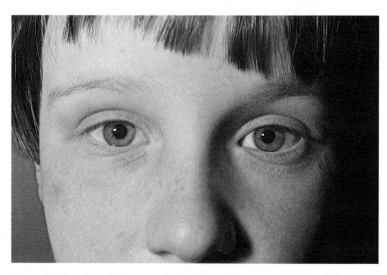

Figure 4.20 **Atopic dermatitis** Girl of 11 with rubbed eyelid eczema and extra infraorbital creases visible.

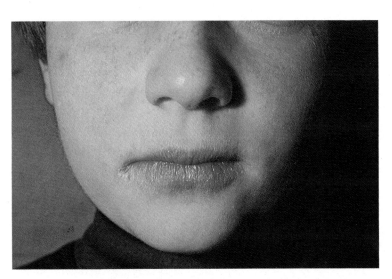

Figure 4.21 **Atopic dermatitis** Same girl with dry lips.

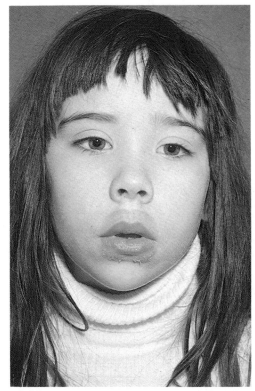

Figure 4.22 **Atopic dermatitis** Licked lips. This child licked her lips frequently and methodically.

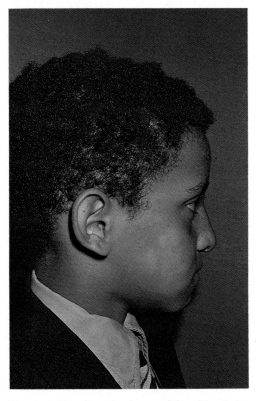

Figure 4.23 **Atopic dermatitis** Pityriasis alba. Note the hypopigmentation over cheeks.

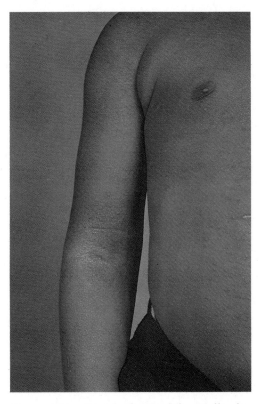

Figure 4.24 **Atopic dermatitis** Follicular papules are shown over right upper limb and abdomen in this 5-year-old Nigerian boy. The cubital fossa also shows dermatitis.

Figure 4.25 **Atopic dermatitis** Same child showing close-up of follicular eczema involving abdominal skin.

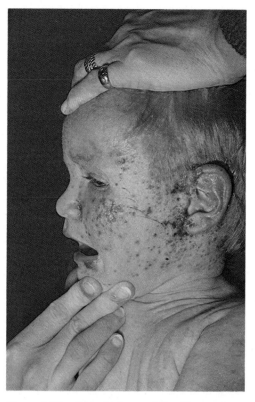

Figure 4.27 **Atopic dermatitis** Eczema herpeticum with bacterial infection also.

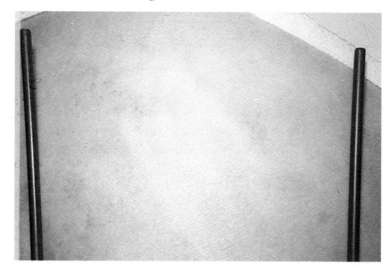

Figure 4.26 **Atopic dermatitis** White dermographism following light trauma.

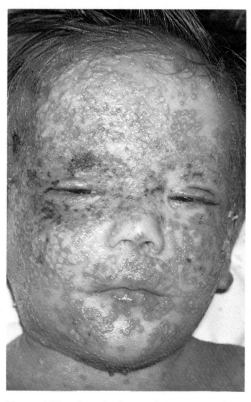

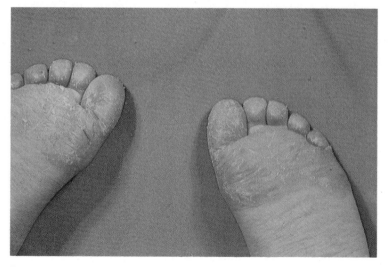

Figure 4.29 **Juvenile plantar dermatosis** Note the dry peeling skin localized to the forefoot in this atopic boy of 7 years.

Figure 4.28 **Atopic dermatitis** Eczema herpeticum. More severe and some typical vesicles can be seen.

eczema, dry cracked lips, lip-licking, and pityriasis alba in which scaling and hypo-pigmented patches appear over the facial skin particularly in dark-skinned individuals. Follicular papules are a prominent feature in the black child with atopic dermatitis.

White dermographism, which is easily elicited over the back, presents as white macular areas when light pressure is applied to the skin. It is due to capillary constriction and is often pronounced in atopic dermatitis.

Contact with herpes simplex sufferers with active cold sores must be avoided because the individual with active or latent eczema may develop a widespread simplex infection termed *eczema herpeticum* and be very ill. Eczema herpeticum is usually a manifestation of primary herpetic infection.

Regarding prognosis, it is true that eczema tends to improve with increasing age, a point one always emphasizes to parents, but it is impossible to prophesy the prognosis in a particular child. Atopic dermatitis affects the individual but influences the whole family and treatment must be directed towards the parents as well as to the child. Occasionally there may be relevant dietary factors and short-term elimination diets and use of soya-based milk substitutes can be worthwhile in such cases. Hypersensitivity to inhaled allergens may also be important. Breast feeding is always to be encouraged, particularly in the first three months of life, and in some cases it may delay the onset of atopic dermatitis.

Topical applications including emollients, bath oils, tar and tar-impregnated bandages, urea cream, and weak steroids are the mainstay of management. Antihistamines in a dose sufficient to allay itching are useful and short-term dosage of adult proportions may be essential if itching is severe.

JUVENILE PLANTAR DERMATOSIS (Figures 4.29, 4.30) is a frictional dermatitis seen frequently in the 0–17-year-old group in which itching and burning occurs over the plantar aspect of the big toe and then spreads to the other toes and the whole forefoot. The heel may be affected but to a lesser degree. The affected forefoot becomes red, glazed, dry, cracked, sore and painful and there is often peeling and bleeding. The child may have difficulty in walking. Toe spaces are notably unaffected. The disorder was first observed in the 1960s and there is little doubt that synthetic footwear with little or absent permeability and poor moisture absorption is an important factor in the aetiology. We believe atopics to be prone to the condition, but it is also common in non-atopics. We carry out patch-testing routinely in this condition but results are consistently negative.

FRICTIONAL LICHENOID DERMATITIS (Figure 4.31) is uncommon and consists of discrete white lichenoid papules occurring over elbows, knees and sometimes backs of hands in children, especially those between 4 and 12 years of age. Most cases are seen in spring and summer and frictional trauma of the exposed areas is considered important.

POMPHOLYX (dyshidrotic eczema) (Figures 4.32, 4.33) is an acute recurrent or a chronic vesicular eruption of unknown cause affecting palms, sides of fingers and soles. Vesicles may sometimes become confluent, forming bullae. Hyperhidrosis is present in some cases. Onset before the age of 10 years is most uncommon. Warm weather and emotional stress often seem to precipitate attacks.

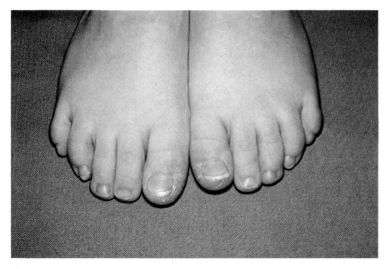

Figure 4.30 **Juvenile plantar dermatosis** Dryness and peeling affecting big toes in another child aged 5 years.

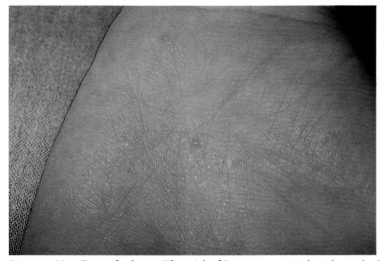

Figure 4.32 **Pompholyx** This girl of 9 years presented with marked over-sweating of fingers and palms. This picture shows just two vesicles over a palm. Lesions are usually more profuse.

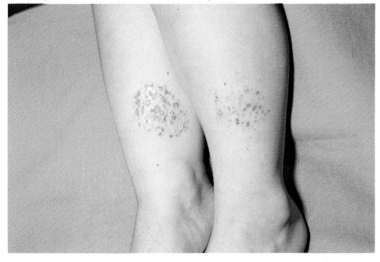

Figure 4.34 **Nummular eczema** Coin-like patches over legs.

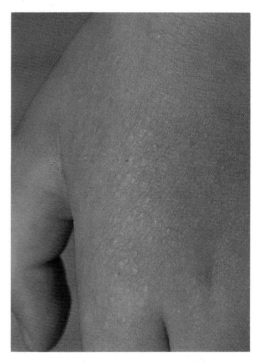

Figure 4.31 **Frictional lichenoid dermatitis** Boy of 8½ years with a 14-month history of plaques of discrete lichenoid papules over backs of hands particularly opposite second and third metacarpals. He also had elbow lesions and had had knee papules. Pruritus was slight. The condition is more common in boys.

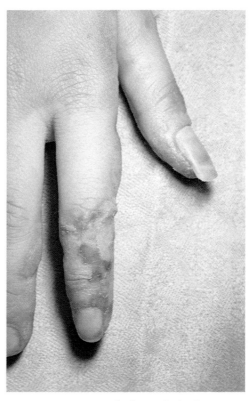

Figure 4.33 **Pompholyx** Girl of 11 years with more severe eczema with bullae visible.

NUMMULAR ECZEMA (Figure 4.34) in children is often a manifestation of atopy. Coin-shaped lesions which tend to be symmetrical are seen primarily over the limbs. Secondary bacterial infection of lesions is common. Nummular eczema has a tendency to be recurrent and chronic.

SEBORRHOEIC DERMATITIS (Figures 4.35–4.37)
The infantile form has been mentioned in Chapter 3. The pubertal child may present with scaling on a background of erythema, between the eyebrows and above the bridge of the nose, over naso-labial folds, involving the ears, and over the trunk. Seborrhoeic dermatitis over the scalp appears as dandruff.

Blepharitis is a form of seborrhoeic dermatitis in which the eyelid margins are red and covered with small white scales. Seborrhoeic dermatitis has a susceptibility to become secondarily infected and is thus often referred to as a flexural infective eczema.

LICHEN STRIATUS (Figures 4.38, 4.39) is an uncommon asymptomatic self-limiting usually unilateral linear dermatitis of unknown origin seen in children and young adults. Lichenoid papules appear usually over a limb and extend in a linear manner over a period of days and weeks. There may be slight scaling associated. Differential diagnosis includes an epidermal naevus, psoriasis and linear lichen planus. Skin biopsy is helpful if the diagnosis of this rather bizarre entity is in doubt.

CONTACT DERMATITIS
Primary irritant dermatitis (Figures 4.40, 4.41) indicating a non-allergic reaction of the skin is most commonly seen as napkin dermatitis (see Chapter 3). The child with atopic dermatitis is prone to irritant dermatitis, but does not show an increased incidence of allergic contact dermatitis. In the infant, a perioral irritant dermatitis is not uncommon from a combination of dribbling saliva, lip-licking and rubbing the area. Uncommonly such a perioral dermatitis may be of allergic type due to certain foods, particularly oranges.

Allergic dermatitis (Figure 4.42) which is a manifestation of delayed hypersensitivity to a contact allergen, is uncommon in children (with the possible exception of poison ivy dermatitis) and particularly in those under the age of 3 years. The eruption always begins at the site of skin contact with the allergen and if contact dermatitis is suspected by the distribution and appearance of skin lesions patch testing should always be performed.

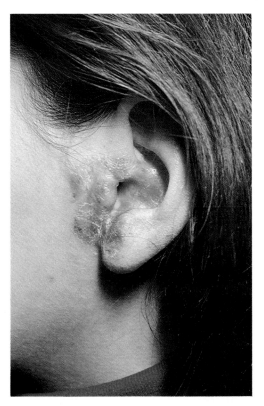

Figure 4.35 **Seborrhoeic dermatitis** Otitis externa.

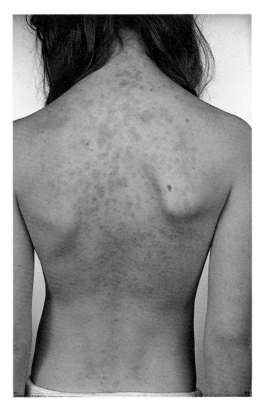

Figure 4.36 **Seborrhoeic dermatitis** Scaling over back.

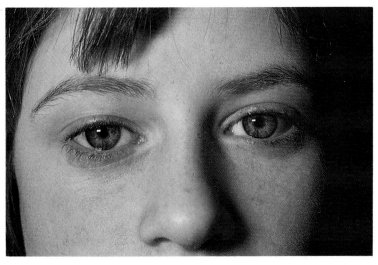

Figure 4.37 **Seborrhoeic dermatitis** Inflamed eyelids (blepharitis).

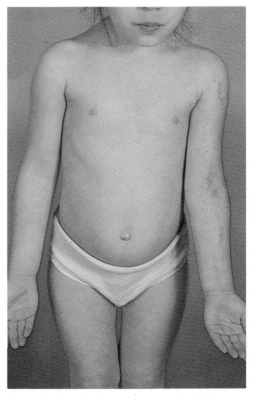

Figure 4.38 **Lichen striatus** Girl of 4 years with a 2-month history of an asymptomatic linear eruption over left upper limb. The condition is more common in females.

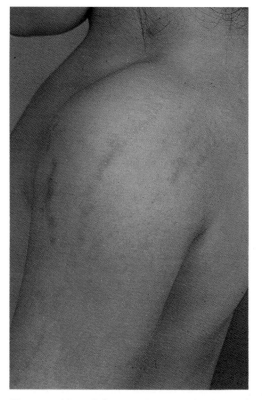

Figure 4.39 **Lichen striatus** Close-up of shoulder and upper arm in same child.

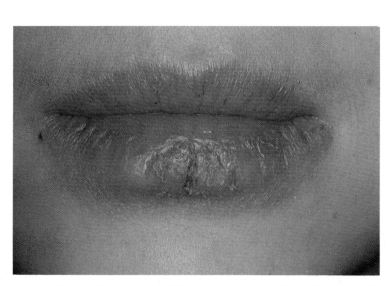

Figure 4.41 **Irritant dermatitis** Saxophone cheilitis. This lower lip dermatitis resulted from contact with the wooden reed mouthpiece of a saxophone.

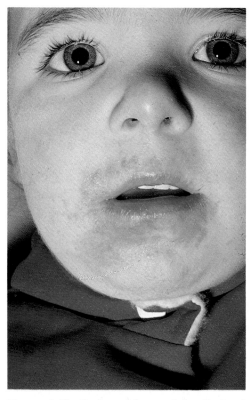

Figure 4.40 **Irritant dermatitis** Perioral dermatitis. Such an eruption could be self-perpetuating if prolonged topical steroid treatment were prescribed.

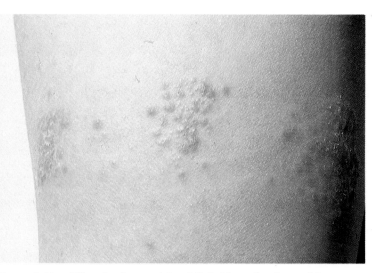

Figure 4.42 **Allergic dermatitis** Nickel bracelet dermatitis.

5
Infections and infestations

BACTERIAL INFECTIONS
Staphylococcal scalded skin syndrome (Figures 5.1, 5.2)
This condition is described in Chapter 3, but it also occurs in children up to the age of 10 although usually in those under 5 years of age.

Impetigo (Figures 5.3–5.6) occurs mainly in children. Its occurrence in the newborn is mentioned in Chapter 3. It is usually due to *Staphylococcus aureus* but may be complicated by streptococcus. It is often associated with poor hygienic conditions and rapidly spreads among members of a household. Flaccid blisters appear, few or many, most commonly over the face, and these quickly dry and crust. Lesions may also be ringed with a crusted edge. In treatment removal of the crusts is important because bacteria are present in the lesions and infected crusts encourage spread. If impetigo is widespread or haemolytic streptococci present, a full course of oral antibiotic is indicated and this may help to prevent the occasional complication of acute glomerulonephritis following streptococcal impetigo. More common than impetigo itself is impetiginization of other conditions such as eczema, scabies, papular urticaria, herpes simplex, and herpes zoster, often encouraged by inappropriate use of topical corticosteroids.

Ecthyma (Figures 5.7, 5.8) is of similar causation to impetigo. Lesions are often multiple and occur particularly over lower limbs. They have adherent crusts with underlying ulceration. Affected children are often debilitated or malnourished.

Cellulitis (Figure 5.9)
Erysipelas is an acute cellulitis due to Group A haemolytic streptococci entering through a break in the skin, usually near the eye, ear, nostril or mouth. High fever is associated with an indurated erythematous oedematous area which is predominantly unilateral at first, but may spread over the face. Intramuscular benzylpenicillin is the treatment of choice.

Low-grade facial cellulitis is much more common and may be recurrent. Sites of entry are as for erysipelas. When attacks of cellulitis are recurrent there is often an underlying

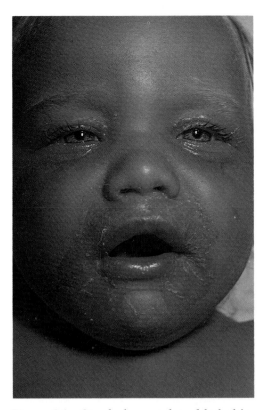

Figure 5.1 Staphylococcal scalded skin syndrome This 1-year-old child showed a generalized erythema. This close-up shows eyelid and perioral involvement.

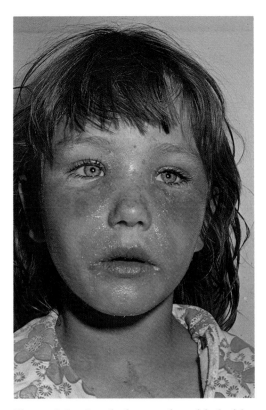

Figure 5.2 Staphylococcal scalded skin syndrome Seven-year-old child who presented with fever and eruption.

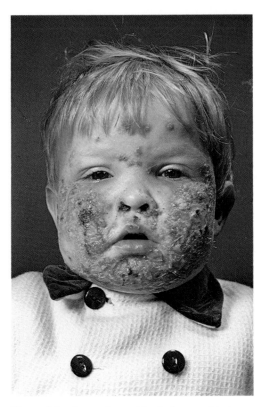

Figure 5.3 Impetigo Typical crusted lesions.

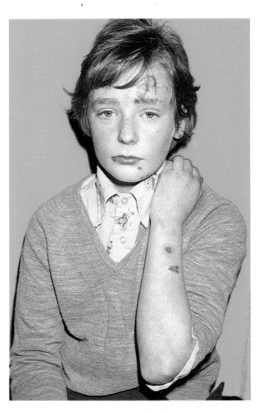

Figure 5.4 Impetigo Facial and forearm lesions.

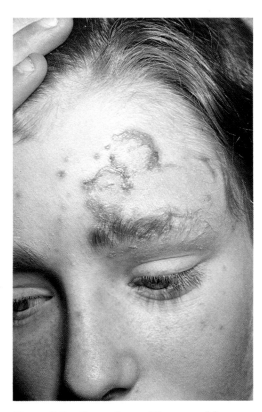

Figure 5.5. **Impetigo**   Close-up of face.

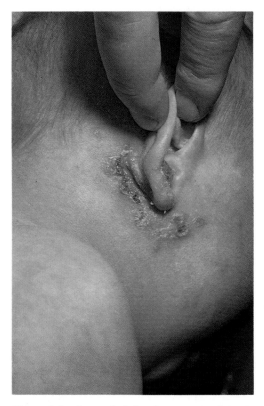

Figure 5.6 **Impetiginized eczema**   Seven-month-old child. Impetigo commonly complicates other skin conditions.

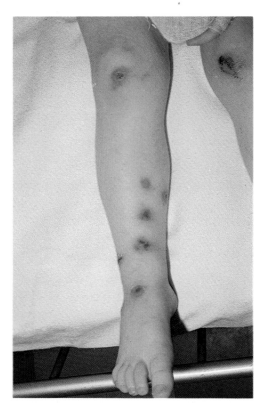

Figure 5.7 **Ecthyma**   Numerous scabbed lesions are shown.

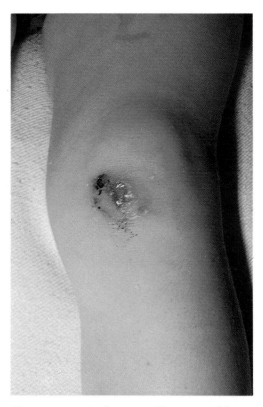

Figure 5.8 **Ecthyma**   Close-up of knee lesion – ulceration under scab.

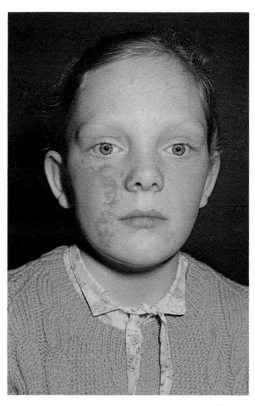

Figure 5.9 **Cellulitis** This shows cellulitis of the right cheek beginning to resolve. She suffered recurrent attacks either unilaterally or bilaterally.

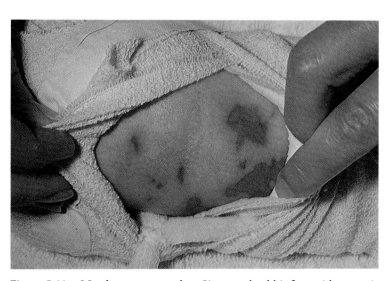

Figure 5.11 **Meningococcaemia** Six-month-old infant with necrotic ischaemic areas of buttocks. Surprisingly, these healed with only minimal scarring.

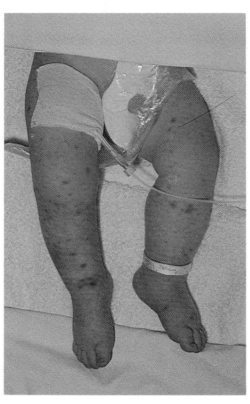

Figure 5.10 **Meningococcaemia** Seven-month-old baby with purpura over legs.

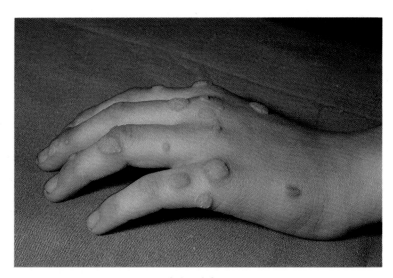

Figure 5.12 **Warts** Typical florid finger warts.

defect of lymph drainage in the affected areas and such patients may show persistent residual lymphoedema associated with tissue fibrosis after recurrent attacks. Although usually due to haemolytic streptococcal infection, cellulitis can be caused by other organisms such as *Staphylococcus aureus*, *Streptococcus pneumoniae*, and *Haemophilus influenzae*.

Meningococcaemia (Figures 5.10, 5.11) may present in infants with purpuric lesions; these are most common over trunk and lower limbs. In severe infections large ecchymotic areas with sharply defined borders may be seen; lesions result from both intravascular coagulation and bacterial damage to blood vessels.

VIRAL INFECTIONS

Warts (Figures 5.12–5.16) are caused by a DNA-containing papova virus which infects and replicates in epidermal cells. Warts, of course, are very common particularly in children and young adults, with fingers and soles being the usual sites, although knees and face are other common sites. In children virtually all warts disappear spontaneously within 3 years and many disappear in months rather than years. Warts are uncommon under the age of 4 years. Patients receiving corticosteroid or cytotoxic therapy and those with atopic dermatitis are more susceptible to the wart virus. Warts are not usually painful but if painful it usually indicates that secondary infection is present or in the case of plantar warts (verrucae) it is the overlying callosity that is painful on pressure over the affected area.

Molluscum contagiosum (Figures 5.17, 5.18) is due to a pox virus and the infection is common in infants and children. Lesions may be single but are usually multiple and appear as small discrete pearly papules with central umbilication; occasionally giant, usually solitary lesions occur. Multiple lesions are common in children with atopic dermatitis and are encouraged by use of topical steroids. The anogenital region, trunk and face are common sites but they can appear anywhere. Parents should be reassured that the lesions are benign and will disappear spontaneously within a year without therapy. Resolution of lesions is sometimes hastened by secondary bacterial infection, but such lesions are more likely to leave residual superficial scarring.

Herpes simplex (Figures 5.19–5.23)

Two antigenic types of herpes virus hominis I and II have been distinguished. Type I causes herpes of the mouth, lips and other non-genital infections and Type II is associated with genital infections.

Neonatal infection often develops in infants of mothers who have active herpes infection of cervix, vulva or perineum. The infant has widespread systemic infection and often herpetic skin lesions. Death occurs in 50% of affected infants. Caesarean section is indicated where the mother has active genital herpes and the membranes have not yet ruptured.

In childhood the primary infection with herpes simplex usually presents as herpetic stomatitis which is usually seen between the ages of 1 and 4 years. It presents as fever with mouth ulceration, often with a few vesicles over the lips, or as a sore throat. Although the condition usually resolves spontaneously over a period of a week or so, symptomatic treatment may be necessary in more severe cases. Although, as mentioned above, genital

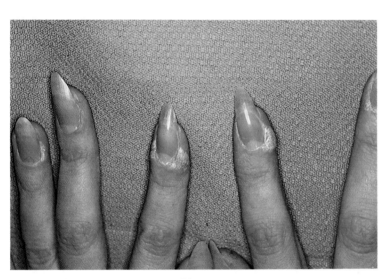

Figure 5.13 **Warts** Periungual lesions.

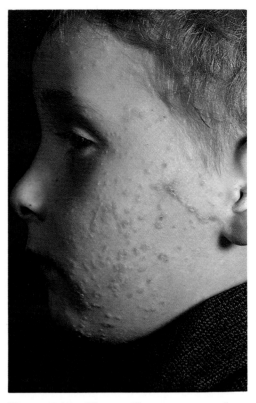

Figure 5.15 **Warts** Flat warts over face. A few are linear, demonstrating the Koebner phenomenon.

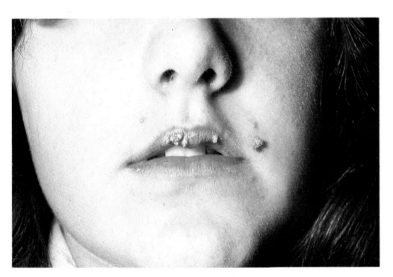

Figure 5.14 **Warts** Lips.

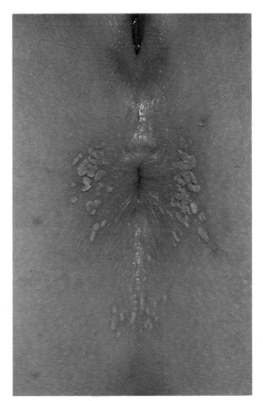

Figure 5.16 **Warts** Perianal.

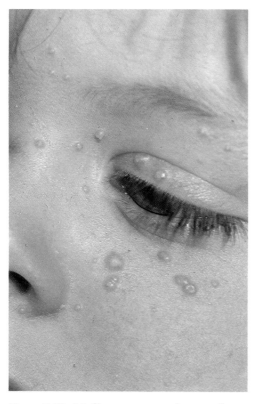

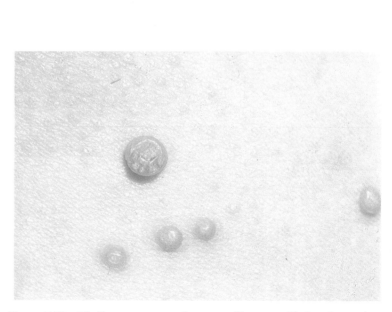

Figure 5.17 **Molluscum contagiosum** Some of the pearly lesions show umbilication.

Figure 5.18 **Molluscum contagiosum** Close-up of lesions in another child.

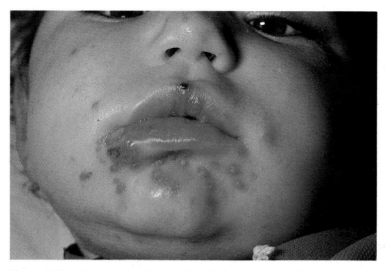

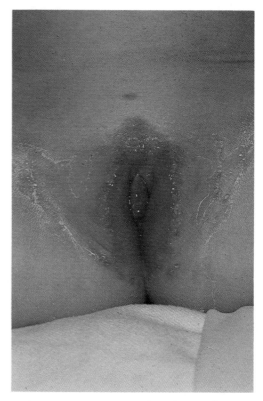

Figure 5.19 **Herpes simplex** This child with primary herpetic stomatitis also shows the common adjacent skin lesions.

Figure 5.20 **Herpes simplex** This 18-month-old child had stomatitis and transferred the infection by touch to produce a vulvo-vaginitis. The area is reddened and exudative and herpetic lesions are visible at the outer edge of the inflamed skin.

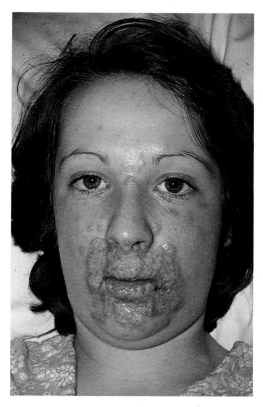

Figure 5.21 **Herpes simplex** Female of 16 with severe primary infection with spread over face. She was not atopic.

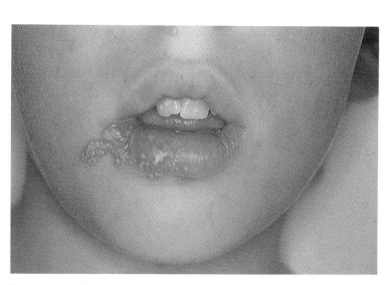

Figure 5.22 **Herpes simplex** Typical lesions in a boy of 10 with secondary simplex infection. The lesions appeared during the course of meningococcal meningitis.

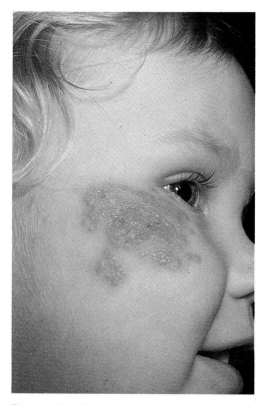

Figure 5.23 **Herpes simplex** Secondary simplex in a boy of 3½ years.

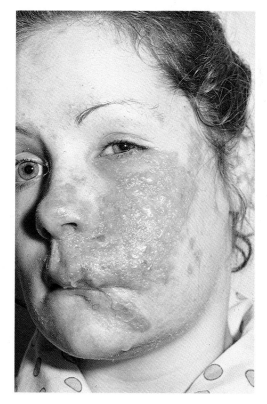

Figure 5.24 **Herpes zoster** Unilateral vesicular eruption over left side of face.

infections are usually caused by Type II virus, female infants are occasionally seen with herpes stomatitis due to Type I virus, who transmit this virus by touch to the vulva, producing a vulvo-vaginitis.

Secondary herpes infection is commonly recurrent and presents in older children as grouped vesicles on a red background, usually over the face. Vesicles burst, dry, and crust within about 10 days. Known precipitating factors are exposure to sun, cold, menstruation and fever.

Herpes zoster (Figure 5.24) is caused by the varicella virus and an attack is due to reactivation of this virus in the individual. The eruption of groups of vesicles on an erythematous background is typically unilateral over one or more dermatomes. Pain, itch or hyperaesthesia in the affected area often precedes the eruption by a few days and groups of vesicles may continue to erupt for a few weeks. Secondary infection of the lesions is common.

Varicella (chicken pox) (Figures 5.25–5.27) spreads by droplets from the upper respiratory tract or by contamination from the discharge from ruptured skin lesions or through contact with herpes zoster. Children under the age of 10 are the usual sufferers. The eruption appears over the trunk on the second day of the illness and then spreads to the face and limbs. Axillae are almost always affected. Macules, papules, vesicles, and pustules are seen in any one area at the same time.

Measles (Figures 5.28, 5.29)
After 3–4 days of the catarrhal stage, the diagnostic Koplik spots disappear while the dark red macular or maculo-papular eruption develops. The rash is first seen behind the ears and at the hair line but within a few hours the whole skin surface becomes affected. As the macules become more numerous they become confluent to produce the characteristic blotchy measles rash. The face is usually the most densely covered area.

Erythema infectiosum (Fifth Disease) (Figure 5.30) is assumed to be due to a virus and small outbreaks of the condition are not uncommon, particularly in the spring. Rose-red papules on the cheeks become confluent giving a 'slapped cheek' appearance. During the next few days, maculo-papules appear over the limbs and trunk, often in a lace-like pattern. The eruption fades within 10 days and symptoms are minimal.

Hand, foot and mouth disease (Figure 5.31) which affects children particularly, has usually been associated with Coxsackie virus A16. The disease is commonly mild, lasting about 7 days with an incubation period of 5–7 days. It presents with a painful stomatitis with superficial small flaccid blisters visible over the buccal mucosa. Similar vesicles occur over hands and feet and a maculo-papular rash may appear over the buttocks. If in close contact whole families are often affected.

FUNGAL INFECTIONS
Candidiasis
Oral candidiasis is common in the newborn and can also affect older children. Patches of adherent white material are seen scattered over the mucous membrane: in the newborn the organism is usually derived from the maternal vagina. Perineal candidiasis may

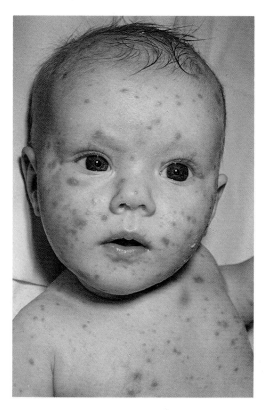

Figure 5.25 **Varicella** Five-month-old infant.

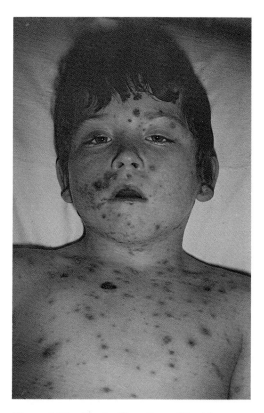

Figure 5.26 **Varicella** Boy of 7 with severe attack.

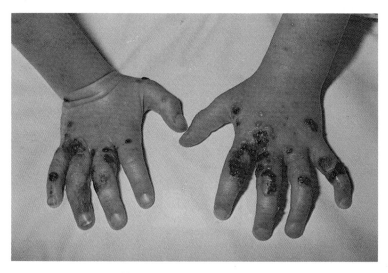

Figure 5.27 **Varicella** Same boy showing hand blisters, some of which are haemorrhagic.

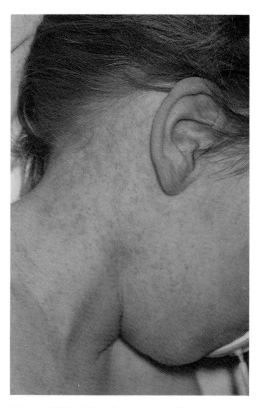

Figure 5.28 **Measles** Boy of 3 with early exanthem behind ear.

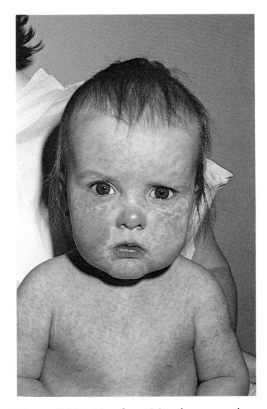

Figure 5.29 **Measles** Macular somewhat haemorrhagic skin lesions. Such lesions are not uncommon and this 1-year-old boy made an excellent recovery.

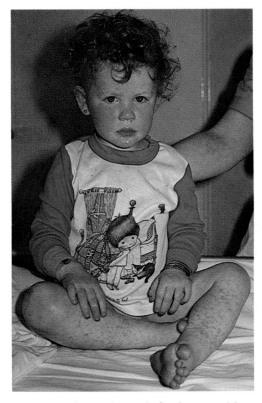

Figure 5.30 **Erythema infectiosum** Note the 'slapped cheek' appearance and the rash over limbs.

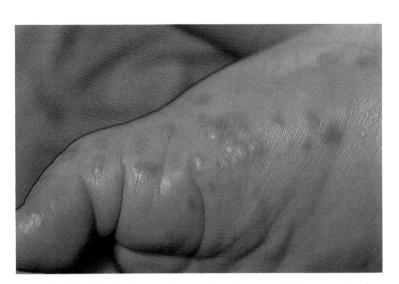

Figure 5.31 **Hand, foot and mouth disease** Vesicles contain clear fluid and show surrounding erythema.

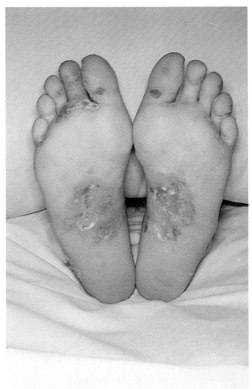

Figure 5.32 **Ringworm** Tinea pedis with forefoot and mid-sole affected and pustulation over mid-soles. Toe space maceration was also present.

follow spread of the organism through the bowel. Napkin area eruptions associated with candidal infection are mentioned in Chapter 3. Chronic mucocutaneous candidiasis is a rare condition with many causes; it affects mouth and nails particularly. Candidal granuloma of the scalp indicates hyperkeratotic areas of candidiasis, in children showing a variety of immunological abnormalities.

Ringworm infection (Figures 5.32–5.38) which may affect hair, skin and nails is important in childhood. Infection is acquired from other humans, animals, or from the soil. Scalp ringworm (tinea capitis) is common but tinea cruris and chronic nail infection (tinea unguium) are rare in children.

Cattle ringworm (*Trichophyton verrucosum*) can give rise to inflammatory red patches covered with pustules (kerion) but ringworm infections from cats and dogs (*Microsporum canis*) produce less marked inflammation and are characterized on the scalp by areas of hair loss and broken off hairs with a varying degree of erythema and scaling. Hairs infected with *Microsporum audouini* or *Microsporum canis* fluoresce green under a Wood's ultraviolet light and this is a useful mass screening procedure. The circular lesions of tinea corporis are easily identified by their active raised red scaling margins. Tinea pedis is commonly seen, manifested by interdigital scaling or acute blister formation. A diagnosis of ringworm can be confirmed by observing fungal filaments in microscopic preparations softened with potassium hydroxide, but culture is required to identify the particular fungus concerned.

PARASITIC INFESTATIONS
Scabies
Human scabies (Figures 5.39–5.44) presents after an incubation period of 2–6 weeks after infestation with the mite, *Sarcoptes scabiei* var. *hominis*, with burrows over the finger and toe spaces, front of wrists, breasts, axillary folds, buttocks, backs of elbows, and penis, but in infants the eruption is often even more widespread, sometimes with firm papules or nodules over the trunk and papules, vesico-papules or pustules over palms and soles. Actual mite infestation over face, neck and in scalp crusts may also be present in the neonate, but in our experience is rare. Excoriations, eczematized and impetiginized lesions are frequent and a secondary sensitization eruption of urticarial type may complicate the infestation. A history of itching in other members of the household is important. If using gamma benzene hexachloride as treatment (see Chapter 3) the possible danger of systemic absorption with prolonged or repeated applications must be remembered.

Animal scabies due to *Sarcoptes scabiei* var. *canis* involves abdomen, lower chest, thighs, forearms and there may be facial lesions. The lesions are weals and papules. It may also be due to *Cheyletiella* species, free-living mites in the coats of cats, dogs and rabbits, and is not uncommon. Pruritus, papules, urticaria, or blisters may be seen, particularly prominent at sites of greatest contact with the animal. In animal scabies lesions usually clear in about 3 weeks if there is no reinfestation. Treatment of the animal source is indicated.

Lice infestation (Figure 5.45) usually presents in children with itching and secondary infection over the nape of the neck. Head lice and nits (egg capsules) will be visible on

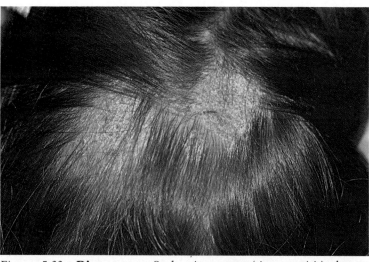

Figure 5.33 **Ringworm** Scalp ringworm (tinea capitis) due to *Microsporum canis* showing two adjacent patches of hair loss, each with scaling.

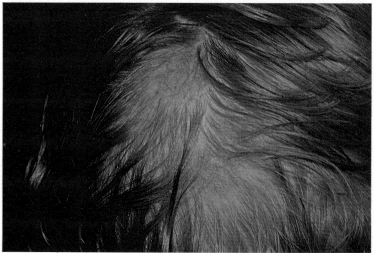

Figure 5.34 **Ringworm** Another child with scalp ringworm due to *Microsporum canis* showing two adjacent less inflammatory patches of alopecia.

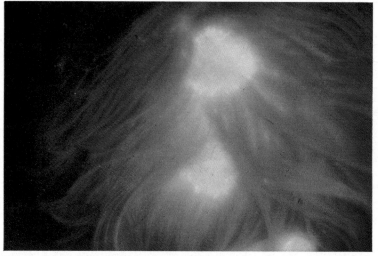

Figure 5.35 **Ringworm** Same child showing fluorescence of these two patches under Wood's light.

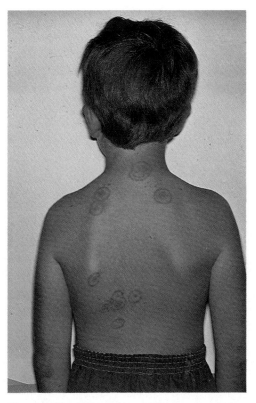

Figure 5.38 **Ringworm** Tinea corporis due to *Microsporum canis*.

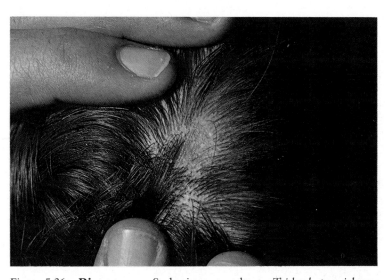

Figure 5.36 **Ringworm** Scalp ringworm due to *Trichophyton violaceum* in a Pakistani female of 3½ years. She had acquired the infection in Pakistan. She presented with multiple small patches of hair loss. Patches were reddened with superficial scaling and an appearance reminiscent of discoid lupus erythematosus.

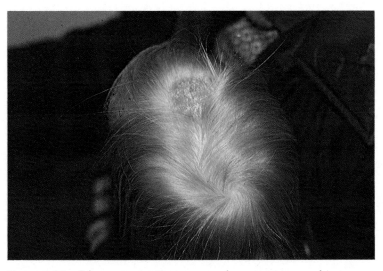

Figure 5.37 **Ringworm** Kerion on scalp appearing as a skin tumour here. The father had active ringworm due to *Trichophyton verrucosum* over the neck.

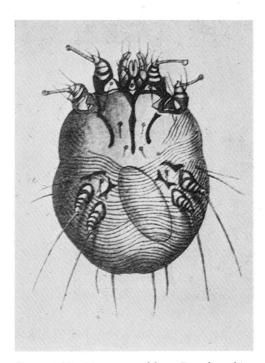

Figure 5.39 **Human scabies** Female scabies mite with egg case *in situ*.

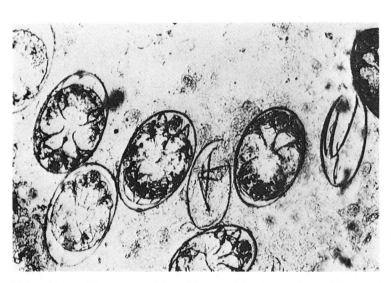

Figure 5.40 **Human scabies** Photograph of scraping of burrow showing numerous larvae and empty egg cases.

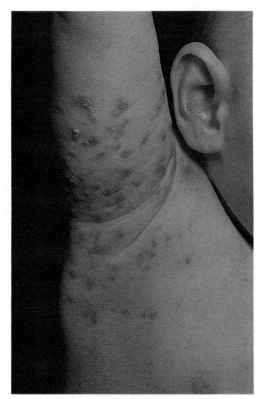

Figure 5.41 **Human scabies** Ten-month-old baby with florid lesions axillae.

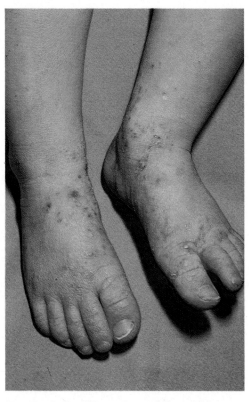

Figure 5.42 **Human scabies** Twenty-month-old infant with ankle and foot lesions.

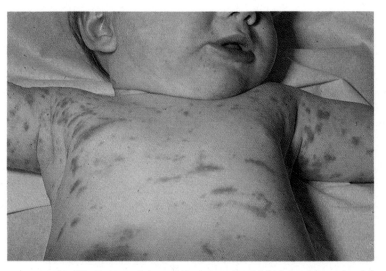

Figure 5.43 **Human scabies** Nine-month old baby with urticarial reaction and eczematization of some lesions. He had had scabies since the age of 4 months.

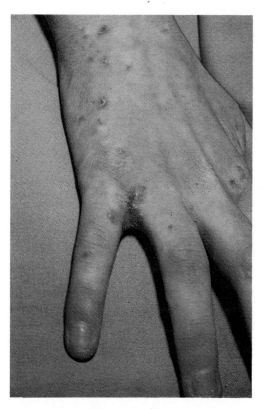

Figure 5.44 **Human scabies** Finger space involvement.

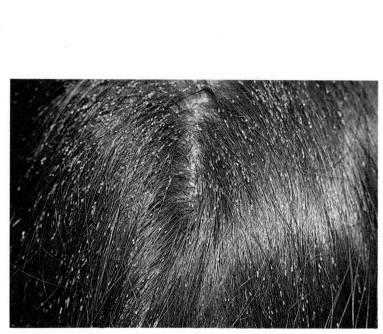

Figure 5.45 **Lice** Head lice (*Pediculosis capitis*) infestation. Numerous nits can be seen on hairs.

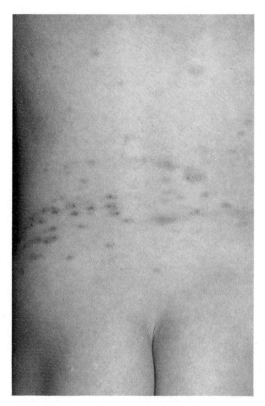

Figure 5.46 **Insect bites** Flea bites are visible over left hip.

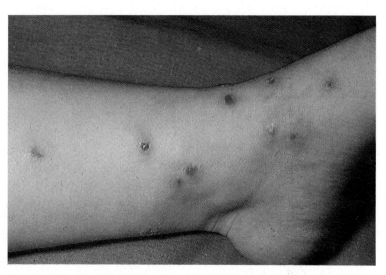

Figure 5.47 **Papular urticaria** Typical site over leg showing vesicles, some secondarily infected.

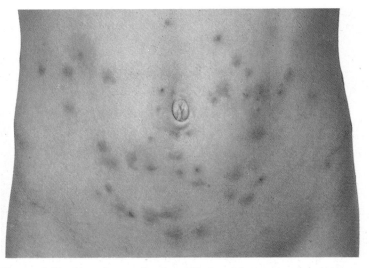

Figure 5.48 **Papular urticaria** Weals and excoriated lesions over trunk.

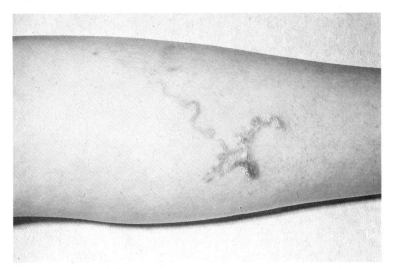

Figure 5.49 **Creeping eruption** The striking serpiginous eruption is well shown.

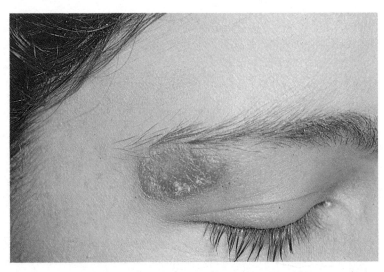

Figure 5.50 **Cutaneous leishmaniasis** Brown granulomatous lesion above right eye. This lesion had first appeared 7 months previously, a few weeks after a holiday in Majorca. It began as a pimple which enlarged, became raised, ulcerated, and scabbed. The lesion was photographed after systemic and during intralesional treatment with sodium stibogluconate. One year after the lesion appeared it was flat with a slightly atrophic centre.

careful examination. All scalps in the household or classroom should be checked and treated if necessary. For routine treatment gamma benzene hexachloride 1% in a shampoo base should be rubbed into the wet scalp, left for 5 minutes, and then rinsed off. The hair is then combed thoroughly and the treatment repeated 1 week later. Alternatively, 0·5% carbaryl shampoo or lotion or 0·5% malathion lotion is recommended. Hair cutting is unnecessary.

Flea bites (Figure 5.46) from human, bird, cat or dog fleas appear in the young as groups of erythematous macular lesions, each with a central punctum. They are often noticed first thing in the morning on awakening.

Papular urticaria (Figures 5.47, 5.48) is more common than actual insect bites in children. It is rare in the first year of life. It represents a hypersensitivity reaction to such a bite from a flea, bed bug, mosquito, or dog louse. Irritation, vesicles, papules, and weals appear over buttocks and lower limbs but distribution may be wider in chronic papular urticaria, and secondary infection of lesions is common. Usually only one child in a family shows the reaction which tends to recur yearly in the summer for a few years.

Creeping eruption (cutaneous larva migrans) (Figure 5.49) is a tortuous linear eruption caused in the majority of cases by larvae of the dog or cat hookworm. Infections are most common in warm, humid and sandy coastal areas of tropical and subtropical regions. The larvae penetrate human skin that has been in contact with contaminated sandy areas and they remain in the skin producing a characteristic serpentine tract.

Cutaneous leishmaniasis (oriental sore) (Figure 5.50) is an infective granuloma of skin and subcutaneous tissues. The infestation is common among inhabitants of the Mediterranean, the Middle East, India and South America and in those who travel to these places. The flagellated protozoon parasite (*Leishmania tropica*) is present in juice aspirated from the spreading edge of a sore. The infection is carried by sandflies (*Phlebotomus papatasii*). The incubation period following the bite varies from weeks to many months. An enlarging irritant nodule appears which forms a sore and scabs: ulceration may occur in weeks or months. Lesions may be single or multiple. Common sites are face, legs and arms. Without treatment, healing with a prominent scar usually takes place within a year. Treatment includes removal of crusts and use of antimonials.

6

Psoriasis and other erythemato-squamous disorders

PSORIASIS (Figures 6.1–6.12) is a common chronic genetically determined condition of unknown cause, and it is seen frequently in children. However, onset before the age of 5 years is unusual and before the age of 2 is rare. In children the most common type is guttate (small spot) psoriasis which appears abruptly, often after a streptococcal tonsillitis or other infection. The small papular lesions have overlying silvery scales. The eruption persists for up to 3 months and resolves spontaneously. However, it is usual for psoriasis to recur within the following 5 years.

The Koebner phenomenon in which lesions appear along the site of skin injury may be seen in active psoriasis. However, it is also found in other conditions such as lichen planus and viral warts.

The plaque type of psoriasis (psoriasis vulgaris) is less common in children and apart from plaques, annular patches of varying size often occur. Psoriatic plaques may be encircled by a clear pale zone, the ring of Woronoff.

Patchy thick scaling areas are typical of scalp psoriasis and when the scales are removed some hair may be lost, but almost always regrows. Pityriasis amiantacea, which can be an early sign of psoriasis, is mentioned in Chapter 10.

Nail changes are seen, particularly in chronic psoriasis, but are unusual in children although onycholysis and pitting may be seen. Pustular psoriasis is rare in children but it should be mentioned as a warning against the increasing use of topical corticosteroids in the treatment of ordinary psoriasis because their use may precipitate the pustular form. Napkin psoriasis has been mentioned in Chapter 3.

As regards topical treatment of psoriasis, bland ointments are recommended for guttate psoriasis. Coal tar-containing applications are useful for both psoriasis vulgaris and scalp psoriasis, coal tar solution can be added to the bath, and dithranol (anthralin) is very effective in the more resistant plaque forms of psoriasis. Ultraviolet light has a beneficial effect in most individuals, but if marked erythema develops with it or with natural sunlight, psoriasis may be provoked.

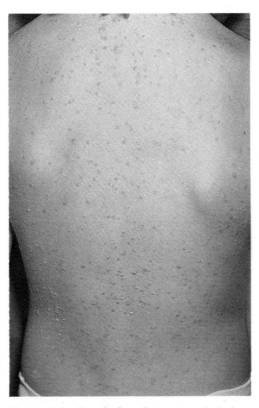

Figure 6.1 **Psoriasis** Guttate psoriasis in a boy of 5½ years.

Figure 6.2 **Psoriasis** Close-up of same patient.

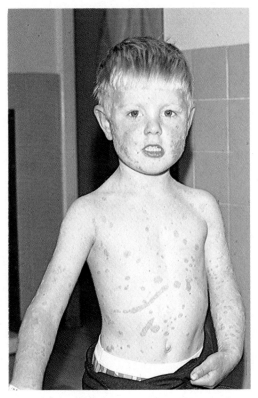

Figure 6.3 **Psoriasis** Boy of 5 showing both guttate and larger lesions and Koebner phenomenon. He also has facial involvement.

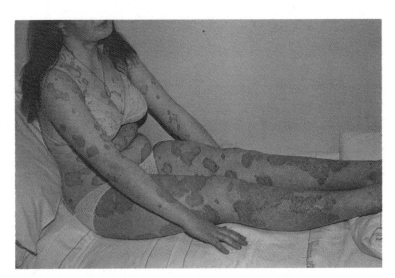

Figure 6.4 **Psoriasis** Widespread plaque type with many annular lesions in a girl of 16.

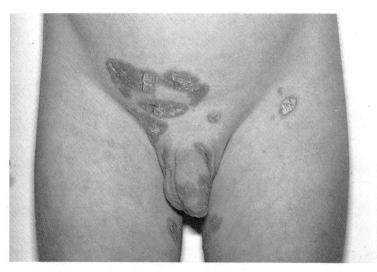

Figure 6.5 **Psoriasis** Note the involvement of penile and scrotal skin.

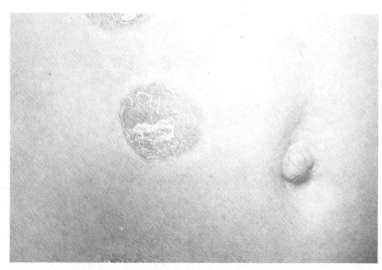

Figure 6.6 **Psoriasis** This girl of 6 had psoriasis localized to the right side of the abdomen. The plaques show the characteristic clear peripheral halo of Woronoff.

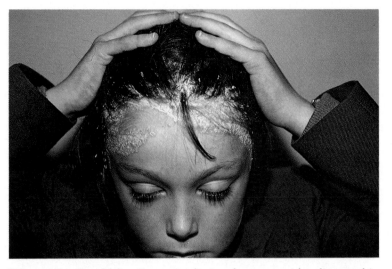

Figure 6.7 **Psoriasis** Severe scalp involvement with adjacent skin affected.

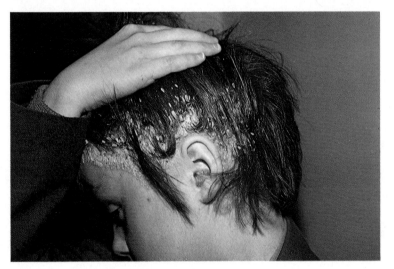

Figure 6.8 **Psoriasis** Same child.

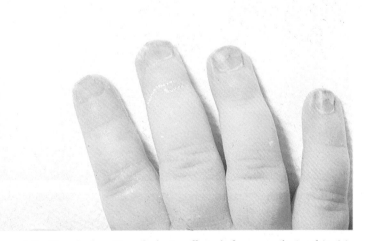

Figure 6.9 **Psoriasis** Onycholysis affected finger nails in this 14-month-old infant with psoriasis. Psoriatic nail changes are unusual in children.

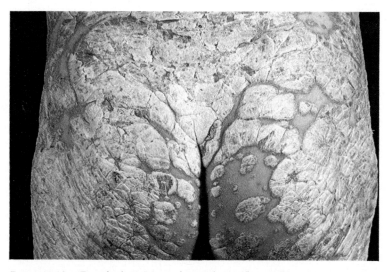

Figure 6.10   **Psoriasis**   Severe buttock involvement.

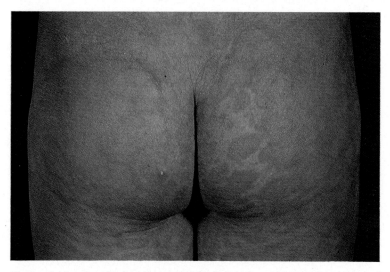

Figure 6.11   **Psoriasis**   Same child 18 days later having been treated with topical dithranol in Lassar's paste only.

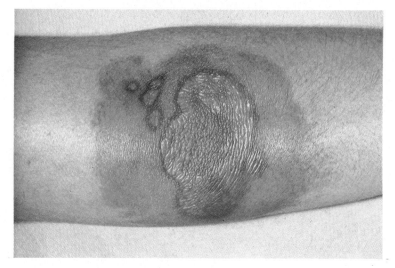

Figure 6.12   **Psoriasis**   Typical dithranol staining over elbow. Such staining clears in a week or so after cessation of treatment.

PITYRIASIS ROSEA (Figures 6.13–6.16) is a presumed but unproven virus infection of 4 to 6 weeks' duration, most commonly seen in children and young adults. The first lesion is termed the herald patch and precedes others by a few days; the rash is typically irritant after a bath. Superficial scaly patches with increased scaling from the centre appear, particularly over the trunk, sometimes noticeably in the line of the ribs over the posterior rib cage. Occasionally, in acute cases, lesions may be papular and even vesicular at first but some more typical scaling lesions can usually be found sooner or later. Purpuric lesions occur occasionally, but once again more typical lesions peeling at their central portion will also be visible. Maximum incidence is in the winter months. If irritation is marked weak topical corticosteroid creams are useful.

PITYRIASIS LICHENOIDES (Figure 6.17) is an uncommon condition of unknown aetiology, mainly seen in adolescents and young adults. Two forms are recognized, acute and chronic. Histopathology indicates a vasculitis affecting capillaries and venules in the upper dermis. The lesions develop in crops and occur mainly on the trunk and inner aspect of arms and thighs. The initial lesion is an inflamed papule which may become vesicular and have a varioliform appearance. This becomes haemorrhagic in some cases and may undergo central necrosis and leave a depressed scar. Alternatively, the lesions may progress to the chronic stage where there is a persistent dark-brown papule with a single adherent mica scale on the surface. Fresh lesions come in crops every few weeks over a long period. It is difficult to give a prognosis in a particular case because the condition may persist for as short a period as 3 months or for as long as 30 years. No treatment is regularly helpful, although a course of ultraviolet light sometimes seems to hasten resolution.

PITYRIASIS RUBRA PILARIS (Figures 6.18–6.21) is a rare condition of unknown cause and without specific treatment. The disorder may present in different ways including a widespread psoriasiform eruption in which small areas of normal appearing skin are visible or with marked hyperkeratosis and orange-red discoloration over palms and soles. Localized patches over knees will show follicular papules with hyper-keratotic plugs giving a rough feel to the skin. Many cases will persist for months or even years, but frequently spontaneous remission does occur.

LICHEN PLANUS (Figure 6.22) is uncommon in children. It is a chronic pruritic papular skin condition in which the papules are violaceous in colour and flat-topped. Fronts of wrists and lower legs are common sites and leg lesions may be hypertrophic. Oral lesions are seen most commonly over the buccal mucosa as white areas in a lacy pattern. Lichen planus is one cause of a scarring alopecia and diffuse longitudinal ridging of the nails or even permanent nail atrophy can occur. Hyperpigmentation often follows resolution of skin lesions and the skin condition usually clears within a year.

Lichen nitidus, although an uncommon disorder, is particularly seen in children and can be considered a variant of lichen planus. It shows histological features identical to lichen planus yet more focal in nature. Small non-irritant flat-toppped papules occur in groups, usually over the trunk.

ACROPUSTULOSIS OF INFANCY (Figures 6.23, 6.24) is a recently described condition that seems to be more common in black infants. It occurs between the ages of 2

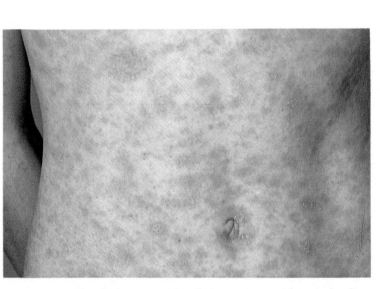

Figure 6.13 **Pityriasis rosea** Many lesions are seen with typical scaling.

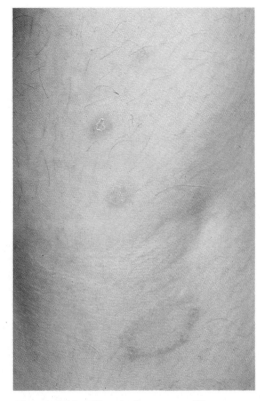

Figure 6.14 **Pityriasis rosea** Close-up to show scaling lesions behind knee.

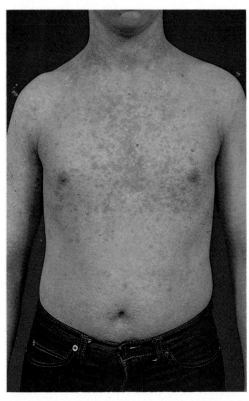

Figure 6.15 **Pityriasis rosea** Boy of 14 with florid eruption. He also had palm and sole lesions and eruption cleared in about 4 weeks.

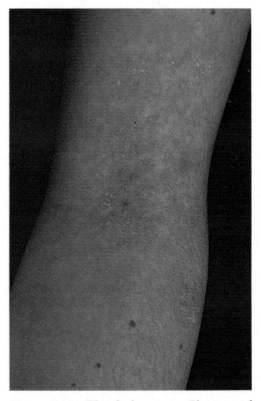

Figure 6.16 **Pityriasis rosea** Close-up of forearm in same child.

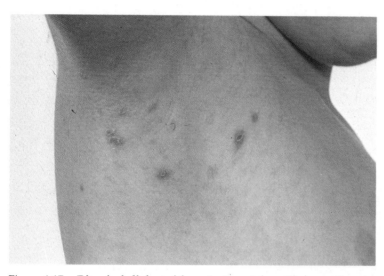

Figure 6.17 **Pityriasis lichenoides** Lesions right axilla, some showing the typical overlying scale.

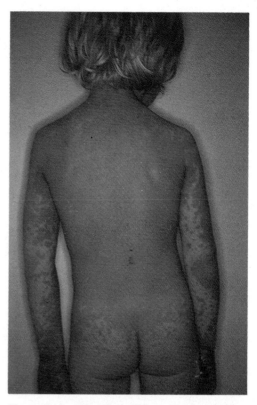

Figure 6.18 **Pityriasis rubra pilaris** Widespread form in a boy of 4½ years. (Courtesy of Professor C. F. H. Vickers)

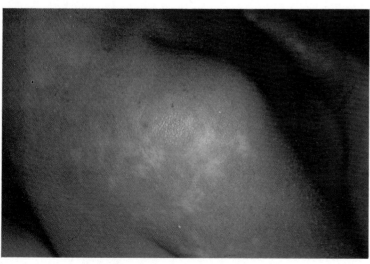

Figure 6.19 **Pityriasis rubra pilaris** Note the areas of normal-appearing skin over the shoulder in same child. (Courtesy of Professor C. F. H. Vickers)

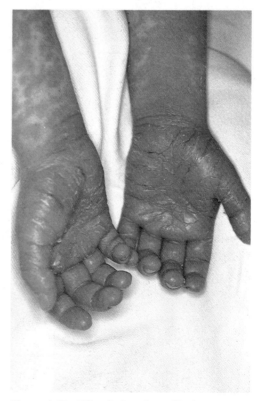

Figure 6.20 **Pityriasis rubra pilaris** Hyperkeratotic fissured palms of same child. (Courtesy of Professor C. F. H. Vickers)

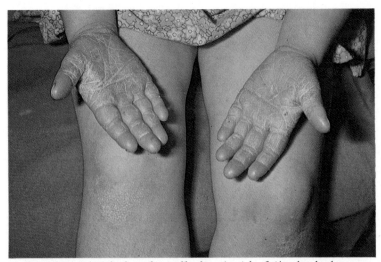

Figure 6.21 **Pityriasis rubra pilaris** A girl of 4½ who had a more localized distribution with involvement of pinnae, alae nasi, and soles, apart from the areas shown.

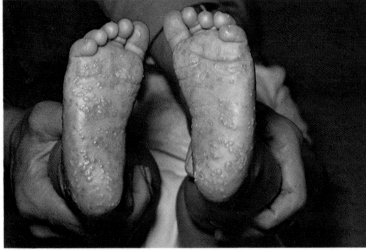

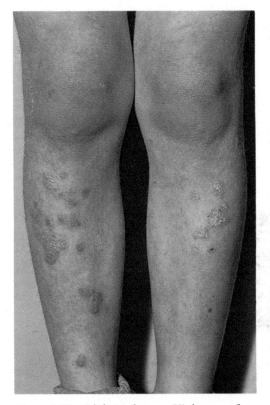

Figure 6.22 **Lichen planus** Violaceous, flat-topped, somewhat hypertrophic shin lesions.

Figure 6.23 **Acropustulosis of infancy** Pustules over sole in a 5-month-old male infant. His mother was of West Indian origin.

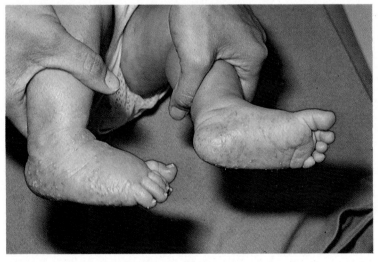

Figure 6.24 **Acropustulosis of infancy** Same infant showing pustules over dorsum foot also.

and 10 months. Crops of pruritic erythematous papules become vesicopustular and appear particularly over palms and soles but sometimes scalp also, a crop appearing over a week or so; then the lesions subside, only to recur a few weeks later. Antihistamines are helpful in reducing pruritus and the condition resolves spontaneously in the first 2–3 years of life. Before diagnosing the condition the much more common scabies must be excluded, while endogenous eczema of pompholyx type should also be considered, although the onset of pompholyx before the age of 10 years is unusual. Histopathology reveals intraepidermal pustules containing polymorphonuclear white cells.

7
Vascular disorders

ERYTHEMA

Erythema nodosum (Figure 7.1) presents with discrete painful red nodules often 1 cm or more in diameter over the shins, and they may become confluent. When it occurs in children streptococcal infections, and much less likely, a primary tuberculous infection, are the usual causes. However, there are very many causes and none is found in about 30% of patients. It is possible that lesions result from the formation or deposition of immune complexes at the site. Apart from the shins, lesions less commonly appear over thighs, arms and even over the face. Attacks last 3–6 weeks and the nodules leave bruise-like discoloration as they resolve. Malaise and fever may precede the development of the nodules and the condition can be recurrent.

Erythema multiforme (Figures 7.2–7.5) is an inflammatory condition with many causes that affects the skin and mucous membranes. Herpes simplex and mycoplasma are well known precipitating causes. Drugs are not an important cause in children. Following herpes simplex, erythema multiforme may appear 1–2 weeks later. The target or iris lesion is a well-known sign and consists of a purple centre surrounded by an erythematous ring; when severe the centre of this target lesion consists of a vesicle or rarely a bulla. Lesions occur over the hands, feet, elbows and knees and there may also be painful ulcers over buccal mucosa and in more severe cases other mucosae. Attacks usually last for 2–3 weeks but may recur. Target lesions are not always present and an erythematous maculo-papular eruption with the characteristic distribution may sometimes occur. The condition is sometimes subdivided into minor and major forms with the most severe bullous form with mucosal involvement being Stevens–Johnson syndrome, a form in which systemic steroids and antibiotics are required.

Toxic erythema (Figure 7.6) is a term used to describe scarlatiniform or morbilliform eruptions due to drugs, virus or bacterial infections. It is distinct from the transient toxic erythema of the newborn. The scarlatiniform eruption consists of a diffuse erythema of acute onset or sometimes an identical eruption localized to areas such as palms and soles. Spontaneous resolution followed by desquamation occurs in 2–3 weeks. Known causes include the exotoxin of the haemolytic streptococcus causing scarlet fever, and drugs. Morbilliform eruptions are usually due to virus infections or drugs. In many cases of toxic erythema no specific cause can be found.

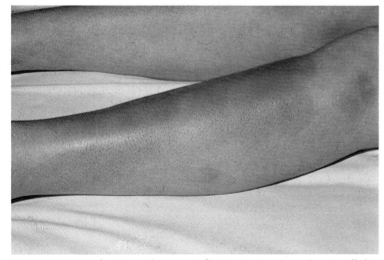

Figure 7.1 **Erythema nodosum** If lesions become confluent, cellulitis may be simulated but erythema nodosum, unlike cellulitis, is usually bilateral and typically excludes the feet.

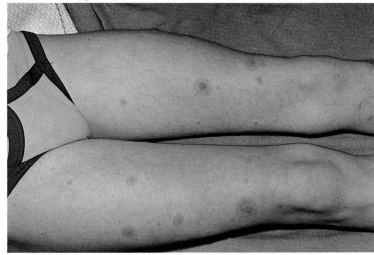

Figure 7.3 **Erythema multiforme** In this boy lesions followed herpes simplex.

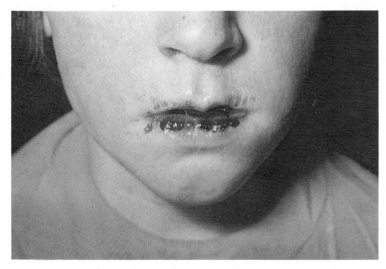

Figure 7.4 **Erythema multiforme** Lip involvement in another child.

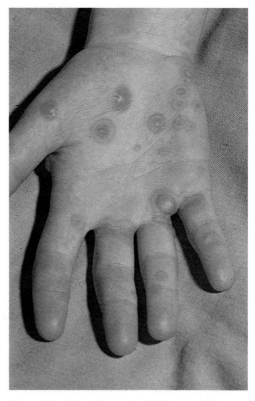

Figure 7.2 **Erythema multiforme** Target-like lesions. Note the blisters at the centre of lesions.

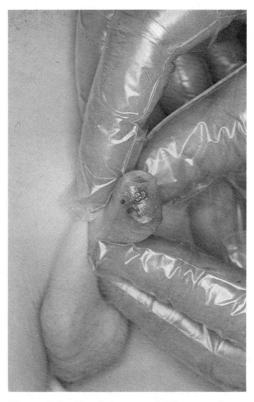

Figure 7.5 **Erythema multiforme** Same boy with involvement of glans penis. Other skin lesions were scanty. Mycoplasma antibody titre showed a diagnostic rise in this patient.

Erythema annulare centrifugum (Figures 7.7, 7.8) is an annular erythema which presents as a small pink papule which extends gradually over days or weeks to form an erythematous ring as the central area flattens and fades. The rash usually occurs over the buttocks, thighs and upper arms, and there may be some itching associated. In children the cause is seldom found. The eruption may come and go over many years.

URTICARIA
Ordinary urticaria (Figures 7.9–7.11) is sometimes referred to as nettle rash or hives and is a transient itchy erythematous eruption characterized by the appearance of flesh-coloured weals. It is due to a local increased permeability of capillaries and small venules. It may be associated with angio-oedema in which swelling of the lips, eyelids, genitalia, tongue or larynx can occur. Giant urticaria refers to the condition when widespread areas of skin are affected. Some residual purpura at lesional sites may occur. Ordinary urticaria as described above is very common and important causes are drugs, food, inhalants, or infections, although many cases are of unknown cause. Acute attacks respond to oral antihistamines and angio-oedema usually responds also, but if threatening the airway, subcutaneous or intramuscular adrenaline injection 1 in 1000, 0·2–0·5 ml, is indicated, and this can be followed if required by intravenous or intramuscular hydrocortisone.

Physical urticaria
There are many types of physical urticaria but we shall mention types more commonly seen.

Dermographism (factitious urticaria) (Figure 7.12) indicates wealing after the skin is firmly stroked or rubbed. It can be observed in at least 5% of normal people. It may begin in childhood and can be so marked as to give rise to considerable pruritus. The wealing tendency with light trauma may persist for months or years.

Cold urticaria is usually idiopathic in children and may be inherited or acquired. The inherited form is autosomal dominant and becomes apparent in infancy with urticaria appearing 30 minutes after exposure to cold and lasting up to 48 hours. The acquired form may appear at any age and may be mild or severe. It is important to warn severely affected patients of the danger of ice-cream, swimming and bathing because histamine is released and if a large area of skin or mucosa is cooled this may be hazardous.

Cholinergic urticaria is a chronic disorder that may be seen in the older child, characterized by distinctive 2–3 mm diameter weals or erythema, precipitated by exercise, heat and emotional stress. The acute eruption usually subsides within 30 minutes.

MASTOCYTOSES (Figures 7.13–7.16) are uncommon conditions in which there are accumulations of mast cells in the skin. Occasionally there may be involvement of other tissues, notably bone. The most common variety of mast cell disease is *urticaria pigmentosa* but *mast cell naevi* appearing as solitary or few nodules which may blister at times may develop in infants and young children, and rarely a *diffuse or erythrodermic cutaneous form occurs*; this latter form is more likely to be associated with internal spread. All three of these childhood forms may show vesicular or bullous variants. It should be noted that the skin of the infant blisters more easily than in older individuals.

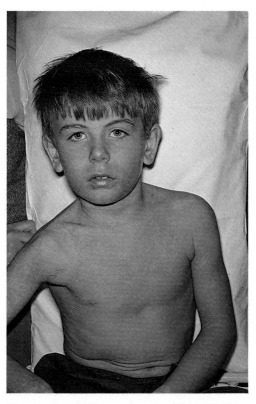

Figure 7.6 **Toxic erythema** This child had a generalized morbilliform eruption followed by peeling, probably of drug cause.

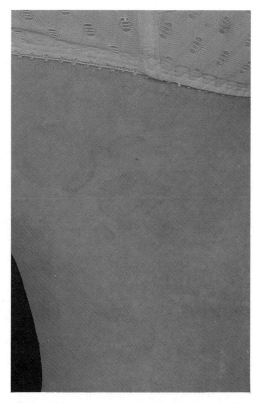

Figure 7.7 **Erythema annulare centrifugum.**

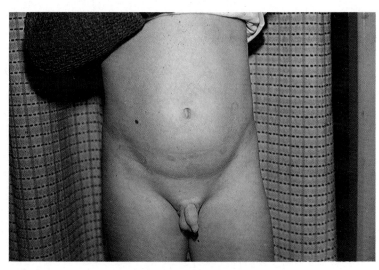

Figure 7.8 **Erythema annulare centrifugum.**

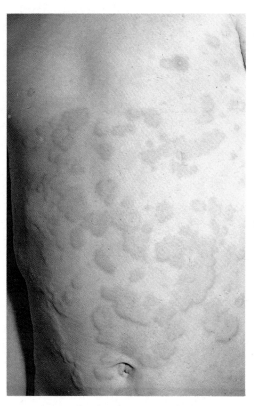

Figure 7.9 **Urticaria** Typical pink weals over trunk.

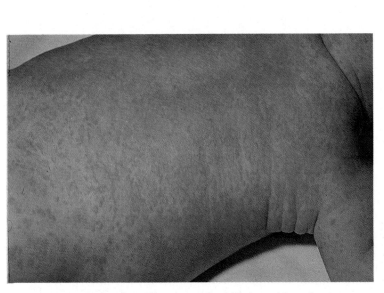

Figure 7.10 **Urticaria** Three-month-old baby with urticaria.

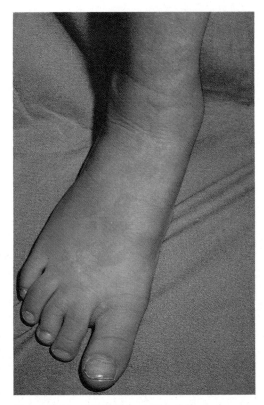

Figure 7.11 **Urticaria** This followed ampicillin in a child of 8 years.

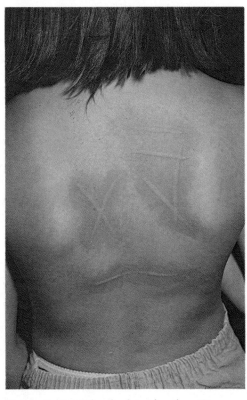

Figure 7.12 **Physical urticaria** Dermographism.

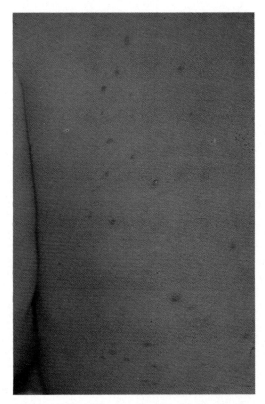

Figure 7.13 **Mastocytosis** Urticaria pigmentosa – papules over trunk.

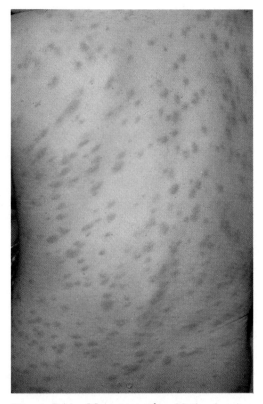

Figure 7.14 **Mastocytosis** Urticaria pigmentosa – more florid example with urticated red–brown lesions.

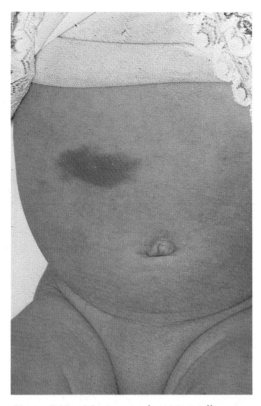

Figure 7.15 **Mastocytosis** Mast cell naevus – brown urticated area over upper abdomen in a 2-month-old infant.

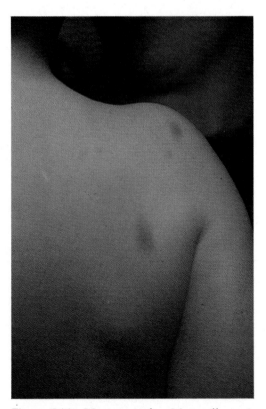

Figure 7.16 **Mastocytosis** Mast cell naevi – this child of 17 months showed about a dozen macular pigmented patches which urticated with rubbing. Now nearly 5 years later the pigmented macules persist but do not urticate.

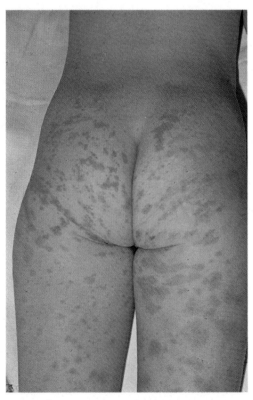

Figure 7.17 **Henoch–Schönlein purpura** Girl of 6 years with purpura of buttocks and lower limbs.

In urticaria pigmentosa lesions may be present at birth or appear in the first 9 months of life. The typical lesion is a small brown–red macule or papule which blanches on pressure and urticates after rubbing. Symptoms may be absent or there may be itching or flushing. Long-standing lesions show pigmentation. The tendency in children is for resolution to occur. Dermographism is commonly present. In most cases of urticaria pigmentosa no family history of the condition is obtained but familial cases suggesting autosomal dominant or recessive inheritance have been described.

PURPURA

Henoch–Schönlein purpura (anaphylactoid purpura) (Figures 7.17–7.20) is an allergic vasculitis and the most common vasculitis seen in children. In about one-third of patients the purpura is preceded by an upper respiratory tract infection. Purpura predominantly over lower limbs and buttocks may be associated with joint pains or with abdominal and renal complications. Lesions may be urticarial initially and in severe cases, purpuric lesions can become necrotic ulcers, particularly over the lower legs. Oedema of face, hands, arms, feet and scrotum is not uncommon. Arthritis develops in over half the patients and knees and ankles are most frequently involved. Abdominal symptoms due to vasculitis of gastro-intestinal vessels present most commonly as colic but occult or frank bleeding, intussusception and vomiting may occur. Renal involvement is usually just a transient microscopic haematuria but a few patients progress to renal failure. The condition usually settles down over a few weeks, but it can be recurrent. Systemic steroids may be indicated in the presence of severe abdominal symptoms.

Idiopathic thrombocytopenic purpura (Figure 7.21) tends to be of acute onset in children. Symptoms other than the tendency to bleed are absent. Bleeding occurs into the skin with petechiae or larger haemorrhages and may occur in any organ. Treatment of acute attacks is by fresh blood transfusions and corticosteroids.

Pigmented purpuric dermatosis (Figures 7.22–7.24) indicates a group of chronic benign conditions of unknown cause characterized by increased capillary fragility or permeability. Histopathology reveals a lymphocytic vasculitis with extravasation of red blood cells and haemosiderin deposition. Clinically dark red or brown patches of purpura and haemosiderin are seen. The lower legs tend to be the site particularly affected. Usually asymptomatic, more widespread forms with pruritus and lichenification due to persistent scratching are sometimes seen. The prognosis in a particular patient is difficult to forecast but the tendency is to chronicity although there is no doubt that some cases do clear within a year.

CHILBLAINS (perniosis) (Figures 7.25–7.28) are localized inflammatory lesions that arise as an abnormal reaction to cold. They occur most commonly in children. They are not commonly seen in homes where there is adequate winter heating. They occur especially on fingers and toes, thighs, nose and ears. Affected areas have a cyanotic appearance and can ulcerate. They may occur over local accumulations of fat such as the wrists of infants; at this site the skin may be swollen and feels cold and sometimes can appear normal in colour. The best treatment of this self-limiting condition is warm, not too tight clothing and adequate home heating.

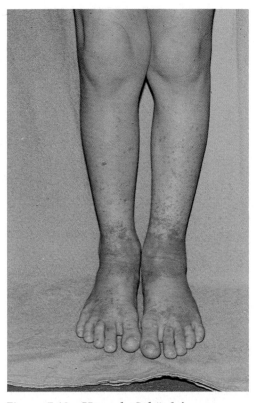

Figure 7.18 **Henoch–Schönlein purpura**
In this child, purpura is marked over the ankles,
which are swollen.

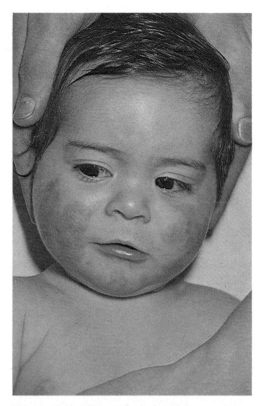

Figure 7.19 **Henoch–Schönlein purpura**
Facial lesions are not uncommon in this disorder.

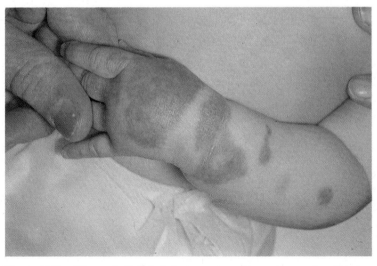

Figure 7.20 **Henoch–Schönlein purpura** Same 6-month-old infant
showing purpura and oedema of distal upper limb.

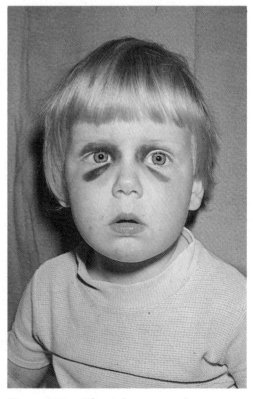

Figure 7.21 **Thrombocytopenic purpura**
Differential diagnosis would include non-
accidental injury.

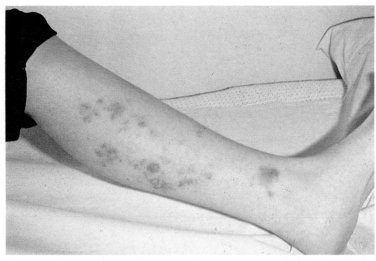

Figure 7.22 **Pigmented purpuric dermatosis** Asymptomatic brown
patches which were localized to the left leg in this boy.

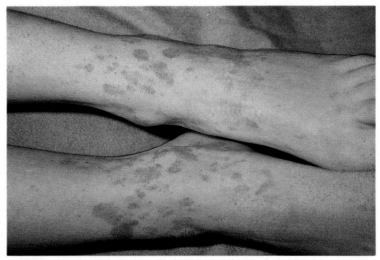

Figure 7.23 **Pigmented purpuric dermatosis** This girl of 12 had
itching purpura with involvement of lower limbs and buttocks and slight
involvement of inner forearms.

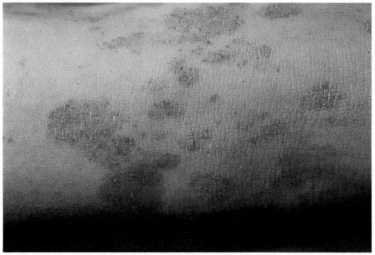

Figure 7.24 **Pigmented purpuric dermatosis** Close-up of anterior
aspect right lower leg. Cayenne pepper spots composed of freshly
extravasated erythrocytes and haemosiderin, and minor lichenification
are visible.

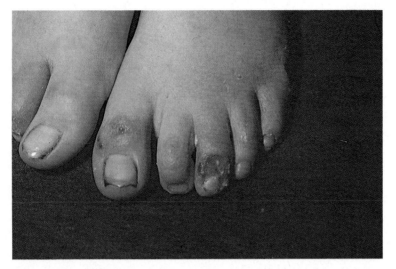

Figure 7.25 **Chilblains** The cyanotic lesions have broken down in this 9-year-old girl.

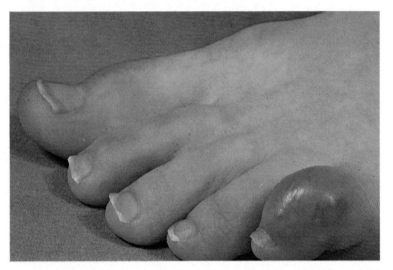

Figure 7.26 **Chilblains** Florid chilblain of little toe in a 13-year-old girl.

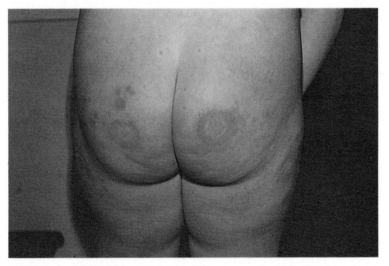

Figure 7.27 **Chilblains** Lesions occurring on a cyanotic background and affecting buttocks and thighs in this obese 8-year-old boy.

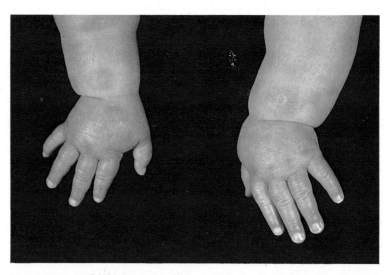

Figure 7.28   **Chilblains**   Swelling and dusky erythema of wrists and hands is well shown in this infant.

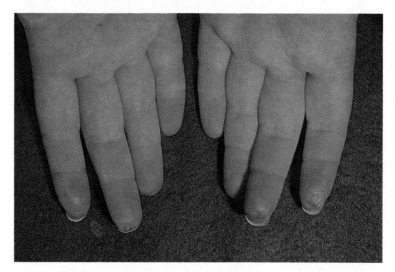

Figure 7.29   **Raynaud's disease**   Girl of 7. Note the cyanotic ischaemic fingertips. She has improved with increasing age.

RAYNAUD'S DISEASE (Figure 7.29) indicates a peripheral vascular disturbance in which there is spasm of the digital arteries producing numbness, tingling, burning and colour changes, in the fingers more often than the toes. The colour changes are phasic, namely pallor, cyanosis and redness. The primary disease is most common in young women but may begin in childhood and is an exaggerated physiological response to cold.

The term *Raynaud's phenomenon* is used to describe the condition when there is an underlying disorder, particularly of connective tissue and especially systemic sclerosis. Some authorities have discarded the term Raynaud's disease because many patients diagnosed as having the disease will in time develop evidence of an underlying condition.

8

Connective tissue disorders

SCLERODERMA

Morphoea (Figures 8.1–8.4), the form of scleroderma localized to the skin, occurs in various forms. In the *common form* there is a localized, slowly enlarging plaque, in which the skin is firm and bound down to underlying tissues. A lesion may begin as a nondescript localized red or purplish area which then becomes indurated. It is commonly seen on the trunk in the form of an oval-shaped area, often with a violaceous zone surrounding it; the latter is present in active lesions. Lesions are single or few in number and tend to resolve spontaneously. There is usually no muscle involvement.

In the *linear form*, which is usually persistent, the sclerosis is limited to one area and may not be extensive. However, if the scalp is affected, with sclerosis of both skin and underlying structures, there can be progression to a facial hemiatrophy. Linear limb lesions may gradually extend to involve the whole limb with atrophy of underlying muscle and bone, and some degree of arrest of growth is likely. If extensive over a lower limb, shortening and limp are inevitable, and amputation due to impaired circulation may, rarely, be necessary.

Progressive systemic sclerosis (Figures 8.5–8.7)

The initial manifestation is commonly Raynaud's phenomenon although weight loss and weakness may also be early symptoms. Visible skin changes begin in the fingers and can remain localized here. The fingers may be swollen initially but then the skin becomes bound down appearing shiny and there may be both hyper- and hypo-pigmentation. Later atrophic changes occur with thinning, telangiectasia, and subcutaneous atrophy. Calcinosis, fingertip ulceration, and the characteristic facies with beaked nose and puckering of mouth can also occur. Linear telangiectases over the posterior nail folds are common. It is important to assess regularly pulmonary, gut and renal function in these patients. The course is unpredictable and spontaneous improvement can occur, but renal and cardiac failure are serious complications.

LICHEN SCLEROSUS ET ATROPHICUS (Figure 8.8) is a condition of unknown cause closely allied to morphoea, but lesions are usually smaller and in females often involve the vulva. It can occur at any age and 90% of cases are female. Well-defined

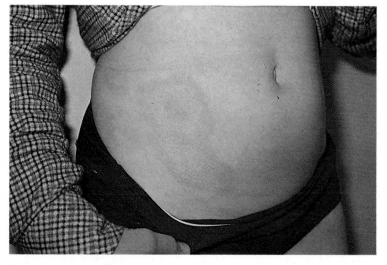

Figure 8.1 **Morphoea** Large patch over abdomen with smaller adjacent patch. Note the active edge of the main lesion.

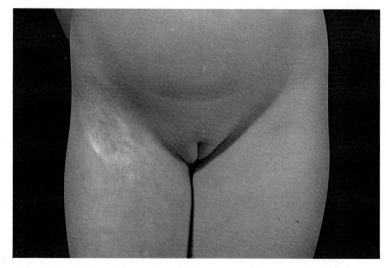

Figure 8.2 **Morphoea** Shiny sclerotic patch over right thigh.

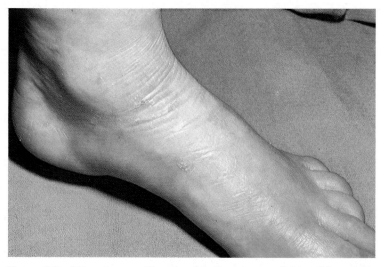

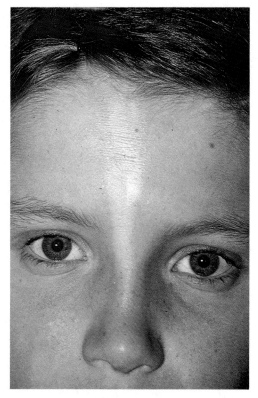

Figure 8.3 **Morphoea** Showing binding down of skin of foot. This child had involvement of the whole lower limb with muscle involvement, limb-shortening, a stiff ankle and contraction at the knee. She was treated with oral penicillamine with no improvement.

Figure 8.4 **Morphoea** Linear morphoea extending from nose to scalp.

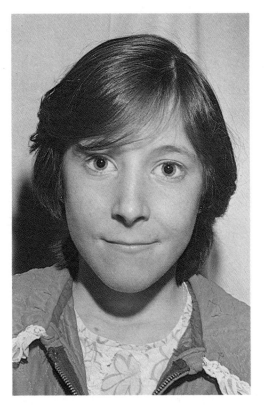

Figure 8.5 **Progressive systemic sclerosis**
Facies of a female aged 13 showing rather
beaked nose. Her general condition had not
worsened when seen 2 years later. (Courtesy of
Dr John Martin)

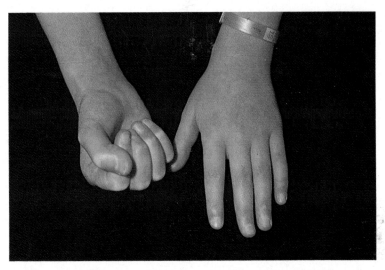

Figure 8.6 **Progressive systemic sclerosis** Same child, illustrating
binding down of skin and restricted movement of fingers.

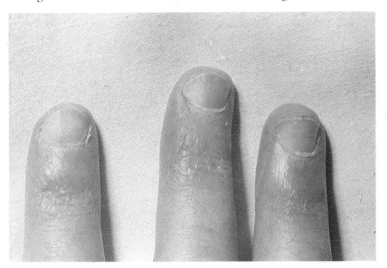

Figure 8.7 **Progressive systemic sclerosis** Same child showing posterior nail fold telangiectasia.

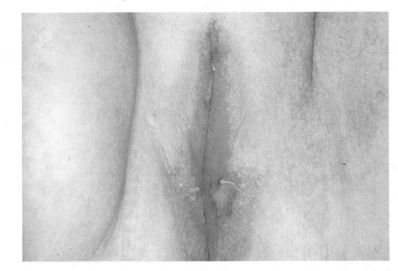

Figure 8.8 **Lichen sclerosus et atrophicus** Girl of 9½ with eroded
skin which followed blistering. Early stage of disorder. This child virtually
resolved completely within 3–4 years of onset.

atrophic changes occur in the skin over the clitoris and of the labia minora and lesions often extend to the perianal region giving a figure-of-eight pattern. Vaginal discharge and pruritus vulvae may be the complaint in children and erythema and quite marked blistering may also be seen. The prognosis is usually good with complete resolution. Topical corticosteroids have a place when blistering occurs or if pruritus is marked.

LUPUS ERYTHEMATOSUS (Figure 8.9) in children is usually of the systemic type and resembles the adult disease clinically and immunologically. Although typically occurring in young women it has been reported in the newborn and may also appear in the second decade. Arthritis, arthralgia, fever and skin eruptions are the most common presenting features. The facial skin eruption may be a widespread erythema with or without oedema, an erythema over the butterfly area of the face or with time, chronic discoid patches. Light sensitivity occurs in about one-third of patients. More widespread eruptions may also occur, livedo reticularis may be present and scalp alopecia which is usually diffuse, may be seen. Treatment depends on the degree of systemic involvement and many children will respond simply to bed rest, salicylates and avoidance of sun exposure.

DERMATOMYOSITIS (Figures 8.10–8.12) is an inflammatory disorder primarily affecting skin and striated muscle but also often involving the gastrointestinal tract. In children, as compared to adults, skin signs tend to be florid and muscle pain and tenderness marked. Any association with malignancy is rare. Girls are affected twice as frequently as boys and the mean age of onset in childhood is about 7 years. Muscle weakness involving the proximal limb muscles and anterior neck muscles is the most common first symptom. The skin eruption consists of violaceous, often somewhat oedematous patches that may enlarge and coalesce and thus come to involve fairly extensive areas of skin. The face is most commonly involved especially the periorbital areas and also the upper chest, elbows, knees, knuckles and around the nails. Calcinosis develops more commonly in children than in adults and occurs in about half the cases in the healing phase and the deposits, which are usually subcutaneous, and often over joints, have a tendency to ulcerate and discharge. Sometimes calcinosis developing in childhood decreases as the child gets older. The main pathological feature of juvenile dermatomyositis is a vasculitis affecting the small arteries and veins of muscle, skin, subcutaneous tissue and gastrointestinal tract. Prognosis is variable and many children recover completely without any specific therapy but oral corticosteroid therapy has a place in some cases.

POLYARTERITIS NODOSA (Figures 8.13, 8.14) is a rare disease at any age. In the systemic disease, eruptions tend to be non-specific and include livedo reticularis, erythemas, urticaria or purpura. In its benign cutaneous form it can affect only the skin, or it may affect skin, skeletal muscles, and peripheral nerves. Clinically cutaneous polyarteritis nodosa presents as nodules, generally on the lower part of the legs. They may be symptomless or extremely painful but they usually resolve spontaneously without scarring, although ulceration can occur. These nodules are associated with livedo reticularis – a physical sign with many causes which signifies capillary and venous stasis in cooled skin. It is the nodulation rather than the livedo that is the hallmark of the cutaneous disease and these nodules show an arteritic histology typical of polyarteritis nodosa.

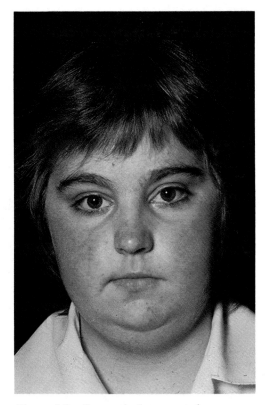

Figure 8.9 **Systemic lupus erythematosus**
This child shows a faint erythema over cheeks
and nose. She was receiving oral corticosteroid
therapy. (Courtesy of Dr Ann Hall)

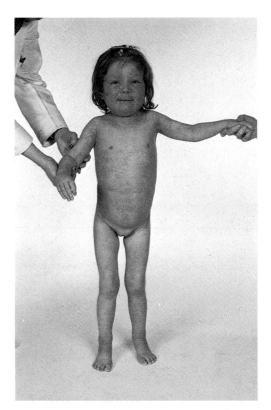

Figure 8.10 **Dermatomyositis** Typical eruption, and muscle wasting in pelvic girdle region
can be seen.

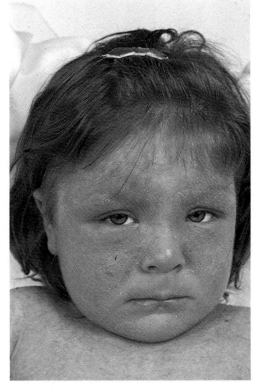

Figure 8.11 **Dermatomyositis** Close-up
of face showing heliotrope colour.

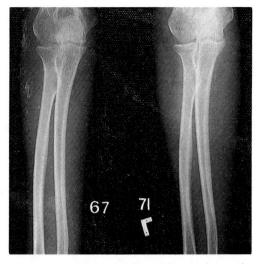

Figure 8.12 **Dermatomyositis** Radiographs
of another child showing some resolution of
calcification over a period of 4 years.

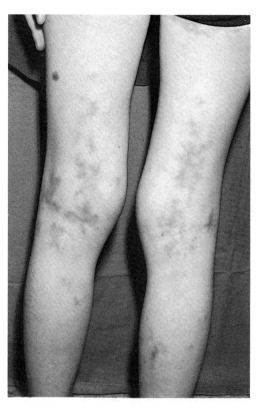

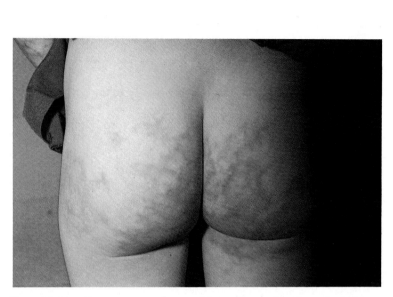

Figure 8.13 **Cutaneous polyarteritis nodosa**
Livedo reticularis. Nodules were palpable both
adjacent to and in the areas of livedo.

Figure 8.14 **Cutaneous polyarteritis nodosa**   Livedo reticularis.

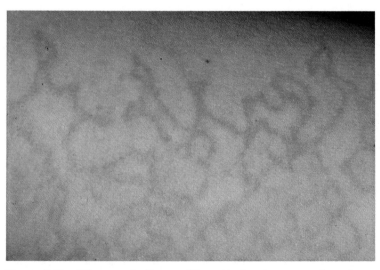

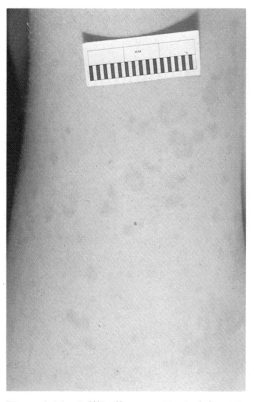

Figure 8.15 **Rheumatic fever**   The reticulated pattern of erythema
marginatum is shown.

Figure 8.16 **Still's disease**   Typical discrete
macular erythematous eruption. (Courtesy of
Dr Ann Hall)

RHEUMATIC FEVER (Figure 8.15)

Although urticaria can occur in rheumatic fever, *erythema marginatum* (erythema annulare rheumaticum) is a distinctive annular erythema which is probably specific for active rheumatic fever but only occurring in 10–20% of cases. It is commonly associated with carditis but its presence does not necessarily imply a poor prognosis. The eruption, which is asymptomatic, first appears on the trunk and consists of flat or slightly raised rings which may be discrete or by enlargement produce a polycyclic or reticulated pattern. Characteristically, lesions fade within a few hours to a few days. Recurrent crops may appear at intervals for many weeks.

RHEUMATOID ARTHRITIS

Still's disease (Figure 8.16)

Rheumatoid arthritis is still referred to as Still's disease in the under-7s, but over the age of 7 the adult pattern of illness is seen (juvenile rheumatoid arthritis). Fever, with a rash and other features such as joint symptoms, hepatosplenomegaly, pericarditis, and weight loss herald the onset. The eruption, which is non-irritant, is maximal at onset and unlike erythema marginatum, it shows no tendency to spread. It is a discrete but extensive erythematous, macular or maculo-papular eruption which is typically fleeting and appears with fever, often in the evenings. There may be an urticarial element.

Juvenile rheumatoid arthritis may be associated with nodules over elbows and small hand joints, which may be tender and can ulcerate. Small vasculitic lesions can develop over the finger tips.

CALCINOSIS CUTIS (Figure 8.17) can be either localized or widespread and be of unknown cause or secondary to metabolic disorders, or to tissue damage in connective tissue disorders.

STRIAE ATROPHICAE (Figure 8.18) are a common finding at puberty and later. Adolescent striae may first develop soon after the appearance of pubic hair. The commonest sites are the lumbosacral region and outer thighs in boys and the thighs, buttocks and breasts in girls. At first pink, raised and weal-like they soon become flat, smooth and bluish in colour. They tend to be transverse and linear and these common adolescent striae get less noticeable with increasing age. They may occur in thin as well as obese individuals.

KELOID (Figure 8.19)

A keloid represents an exaggerated connective tissue response to skin injury. Black persons and other darker-skinned individuals are more susceptible and the tendency is often familial. Keloids are pink, smooth, rubbery and they tend to increase in size long after healing has taken place. They tend to proliferate beyond the area of the original wound. Keloids are relatively common after varicella but usually follow only one or two of many apparently identical lesions.

HYPERTROPHIC SCARS (Figure 8.20), on the other hand, tend to stay within the margins of the lesion. Although fresh scars are often hypertrophic, with passage of time and patience, unlike keloids, they contract and become less apparent. It is important to mention this to parents following scalds, for instance, for often in children the most unsightly scars will flatten spontaneously within a few years.

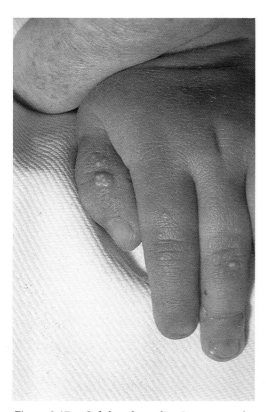

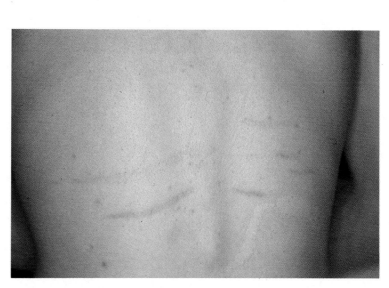

Figure 8.17 **Calcinosis cutis** Seven-month-old male with localized calcinosis of unknown cause.

Figure 8.18 **Striae atrophicae** If looked for they are a common, normal finding in older children. Illustrated here are recently appeared transverse lesions which will flatten later.

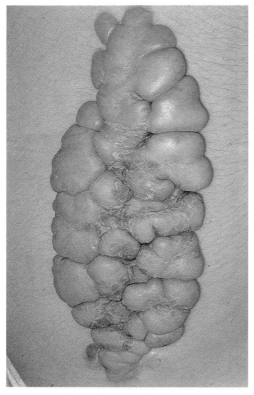

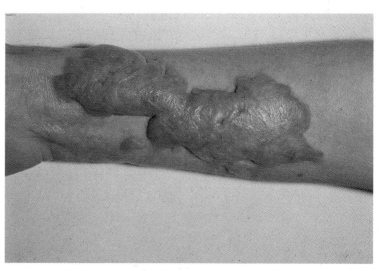

Figure 8.19 **Keloid** This upper thigh lesion followed a hip operation for congenital dislocation.

Figure 8.20 **Hypertrophic scar** The forearm was scalded by steam from a kettle 6 months previously in this 8-year-old boy. Much spontaneous flattening would be expected within the next few years and there was visible improvement 6 months after this picture was taken.

9
Bullous dermatoses

Mechano-bullous diseases

The mechano-bullous diseases are a group of inherited non-inflammatory disorders in which blisters and erosions occur with mechanical, often minor, trauma. They were previously grouped together under the term *epidermolysis bullosa*. However, as a result of ultra-structural studies it is clear that in the scarring, so-called dystrophic forms, pathology occurs beneath the basement membrane so that these scarring conditions are now commonly referred to as *dermolytic bullous dermatosis*.

EPIDERMOLYSIS BULLOSA
Epidermolysis bullosa simplex (Figures 9.1–9.3) is inherited as an autosomal dominant. The onset is usually within the first few months of life although erosions due to skin trauma at the time of birth can be present. Blisters vary in size and rapidly become tense with clear fluid. The condition tends to be worse in warm weather. Mucous membranes are rarely affected. Secondary bacterial infection of blisters is common, but healing without scarring follows. In this condition improvement often occurs with increasing age and protection of the skin from mechanical trauma is the mainstay of management.

Recurrent bullous eruption of the hands and feet (Cockayne's disease) (Figure 9.4) is a mild non-scarring autosomal dominant disorder which usually appears in early childhood, but may present in early adult life. Blisters appear, particularly over the soles, but the sides of the fingers may be affected. Trauma from walking usually precipitates the blisters which occur particularly in warm weather. Epidermolysis occurs in the basal and suprabasal cells of the epidermis in this and the simplex form.

Epidermolysis bullosa hereditaria letalis (Herlitz disease)
In this severe autosomal recessive condition which is frequently lethal in infancy, there is separation between the basement membrane and the basal cell plasma membrane and it is thus more appropriately termed *junctional bullous epidermatosis*. There is severe skin and mucosal involvement, nails and teeth become dystrophic, and unlike epidermolysis

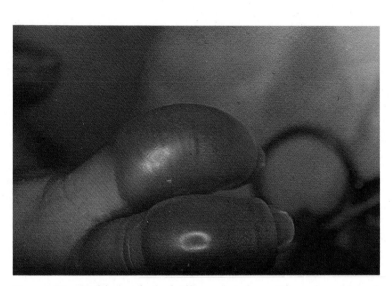

Figure 9.1 **Epidermolysis bullosa simplex** Three-day-old male with blisters over digits.

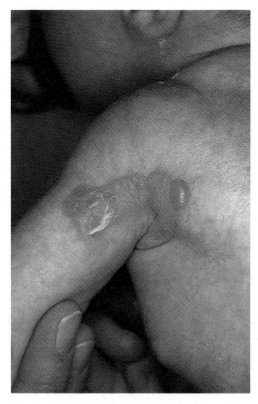

Figure 9.2 **Epidermolysis bullosa simplex** Same child at 19 days.

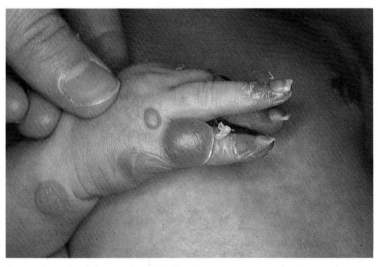

Figure 9.3 **Epidermolysis bullosa simplex** Same child at 19 days showing both blisters and healing.

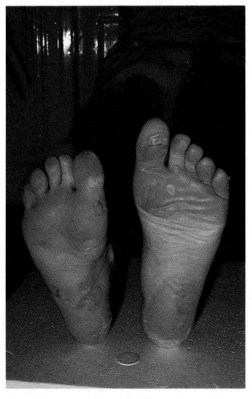

Figure 9.4 **Cockayne's disease** Involving soles only in this girl. She deroofed large blisters with scissors herself. Condition first appeared at age of 17.

bullosa simplex, eroded areas do not heal rapidly. Blisters may be haemorrhagic and are frequently secondarily infected. Genetic counselling is important.

DERMOLYTIC BULLOUS DERMATOSIS (dystrophic epidermolysis bullosa)
Autosomal dominant form (Figures 9.5–9.7)
In this mild form blisters heal leaving superficial discoloured scars particularly over hands, feet, elbows and knees. Nails may be dystrophic and milia are a common finding at the sites of healed blisters.

Autosomal recessive form (Figures 9.8, 9.9)
This severe scarring form appears usually at birth with minor trauma producing blistering and separation of epidermis. Mucous membranes are affected and mouth blisters and erosions, which are sometimes haemorrhagic, are common. Pharyngeal and oesophageal involvement may produce strictures. Hands and feet are particularly affected and healing of these deeper blisters can produce syndactyly, requiring plastic surgery at a later date. Nails are dystrophic and milia in scarred areas are usual. This is a severe crippling form of disease and genetic counselling should be offered to parents of such children. Systemic steroid therapy can be of help to these patients but will affect growth and give rise to other toxic effects in the dosage required. More recently, phenytoin (diphenylhydantoin) a collagenase inhibitor, has been found to be effective in some patients, being prescribed because of evidence of increased collagenase in both blistered and non-blistered areas of skin. It should be noted that phenytoin also has side-effects.

Chronic inflammatory conditions

CHRONIC BULLOUS DERMATOSIS OF CHILDHOOD (linear IgA dermatosis of childhood) (Figures 9.10–9.13) is probably the most frequently seen of the three rare conditions to be mentioned. It usually begins before the age of 6 years and presents with tense bullae of varying size, some haemorrhagic, arising on normal or erythematous skin. The lower half of the trunk, genitalia, and lower limbs are most commonly affected sites. Pruritus may or may not be present. Blisters often occur in small ringed patterns. Histopathology reveals a subepidermal bulla with a variable dermal infiltrate. Direct immunofluorescence may be negative but will usually demonstrate linear IgA deposition along the basement membrane. A circulating IgA basement membrane zone antibody is also present in up to 80% of cases. The condition is subject to remissions and tends to clear spontaneously within 2–3 years. The disease may represent a childhood equivalent of linear IgA dermatosis of adults. Sulphapyridine may be helpful in therapy.

DERMATITIS HERPETIFORMIS (Figures 9.14, 9.15) in childhood is the same as the adult condition, but it has an age of onset from 6 to 11 years. Grouped vesicles and urticated papules occur. Lesions are scattered over trunk and limbs, particularly knees, elbows, natal cleft, buttocks, and scapular areas. Histopathology reveals a subepidermal bulla with microabscesses at the tips of the dermal papillae. Immunofluorescent studies will show a granular IgA deposition at the dermoepidermal junction especially in dermal papillae in uninvolved skin. C_3 may also be present.

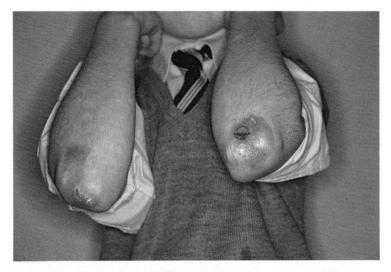

Figure 9.5 **Dermolytic bullous dermatosis** Autosomal dominant form in boy aged 12, showing scarring over elbows.

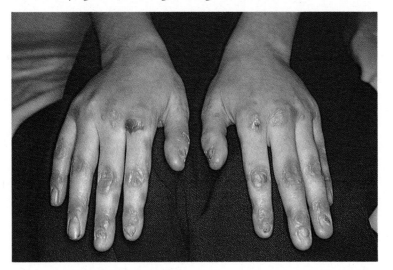

Figure 9.6 **Dermolytic bullous dermatosis** Same child showing scarring, erosions, and dystrophic nails.

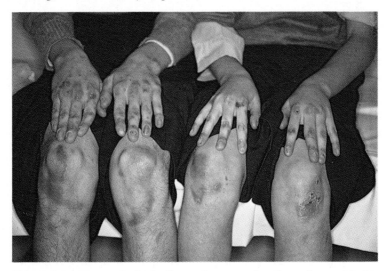

Figure 9.7 **Dermolytic bullous dermatosis** Same boy with his affected 15-year-old brother.

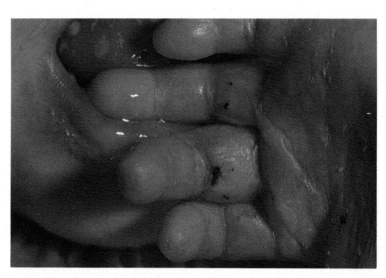

Figure 9.8 **Dermolytic bullous dermatosis** Early stage of autosomal recessive form in a severely affected female infant who was receiving systemic steroid therapy. She shows scarring of fingers and hand with visible loss of epidermal ridges, mouth ulceration and oral candidiasis.

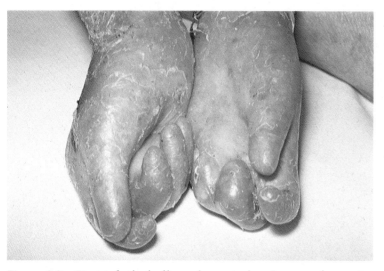

Figure 9.9 **Dermolytic bullous dermatosis** Autosomal recessive form showing syndactyly and severe deformity in another child.

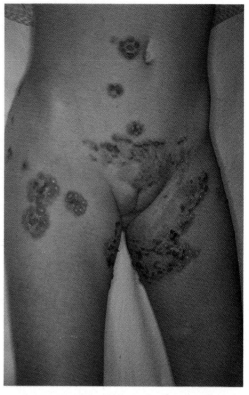

Figure 9.10 **Chronic bullous dermatosis of childhood** The rosettes of blisters are particularly well shown over the right thigh. (Courtesy of Dr T. W. Stewart)

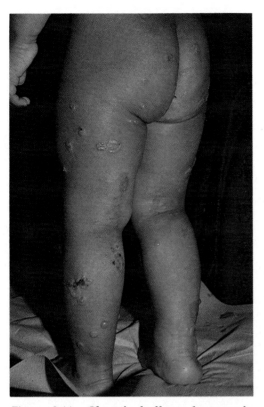

Figure 9.11 **Chronic bullous dermatosis of childhood** Dark-skinned child with same condition.

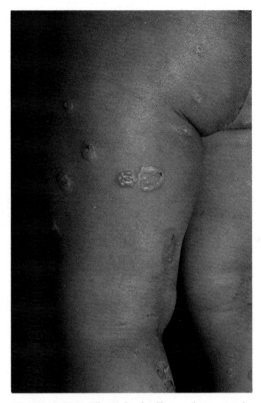

Figure 9.12 **Chronic bullous dermatosis of childhood** Close-up of left posterior thigh lesions.

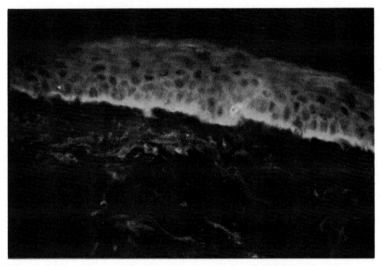

Figure 9.13 **Chronic bullous dermatosis of childhood** Immuno-fluorescence showing linear deposition of IgA. (Courtesy of Dr S. S. Bleehen)

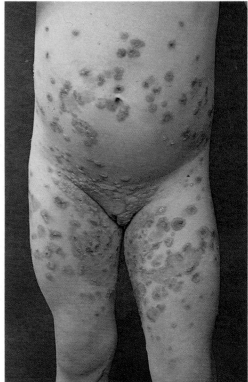

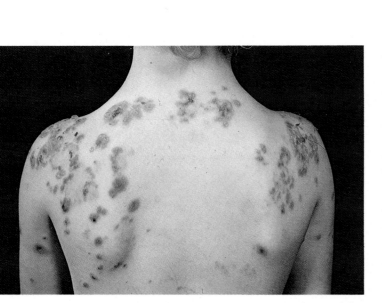

Figure 9.14 **Dermatitis herpetiformis** Typical distribution over scapulae.

Figure 9.15 **Dermatitis herpetiformis** Same child.

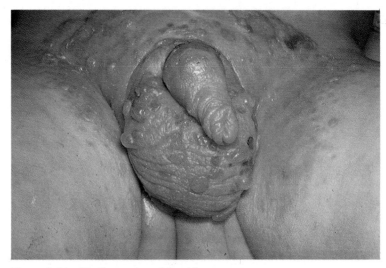

Figure 9.16 **Bullous pemphigoid.**

The majority of patients with dermatitis herpetiformis have an enteropathy, demonstrated by jejunal biopsy, identical to that of coeliac disease. Treatment with a gluten-free diet in such patients will produce improvement in both skin and bowel, but skin improvement may take many months of strict dieting to be obvious. Dapsone (diaminodiphenyl sulphone) also is usually given initially, in a dosage of 25–50 mg a day in children, if the degree of itching is severe. It should be noted that dapsone does have side-effects including haemolysis. Most cases of dermatitis herpetiformis persist into adult life, but periods of remission are common.

BULLOUS PEMPHIGOID (Figure 9.16) in children appears in the under-6 age group. Crops of tense bullae which may be blood-stained, occur on normal or erythematous skin especially over the face, and genito-crural regions, and limbs. It is not pruritic. The subepidermal bullae may be accompanied by a mostly eosinophilic dermal infiltrate. Mucous membranes may be affected. Direct immunofluorescence shows linear basement membrane staining for IgG in lesional skin and IgA, IgM and C_3 may also be present. Indirect immunofluorescence can be used to demonstrate a circulating IgG antibody against basement membrane. Treatment at the present time in children is usually with oral corticosteroids. The condition tends to be self-limiting and usually clears before puberty.

Other blistering disorders will be found in other sections, including Chapters 2, 3, 5 and 7.

10
Hair and nails

Hair

ALOPECIA

Hereditary diffuse hair loss (Figures 10.1, 10.2) whenever occurring by itself is usually an autosomal dominant trait and eyebrows and eyelashes may be affected as well as the scalp. It is usually permanent. However, hypotrichosis is more commonly only one component in many genodermatoses and some of these such as anhidrotic and hidrotic ectodermal dysplasia, Rothmund–Thomson syndrome, focal dermal hypoplasia and acrodermatitis enteropathica are mentioned in Chapter 2.

Alopecia areata (Figures 10.3, 10.4) is the most common form of hair loss in women and children, the male type of androgenetic alopecia being more common in adult males. Any age group can be affected. No specific cause has been found, but in 30–40% of patients there is a family history of the condition. Usually one or two patches of complete hair loss appear over the scalp, although any part of the body may be affected. Early patches, in children particularly, may show an irregular outline. Rarely hair may be lost from the whole of the scalp (alopecia totalis) or even the whole body (alopecia universalis). The condition has some tendency to be recurrent. In the active phase pathognomonic broken-off hairs, termed exclamation mark hairs, are seen particularly at the margins of the area of hair loss. The prognosis is good when there are few patches of hair loss, with likely regrowth in 6–12 months, but the more extensive the loss the more guarded should be the prognosis. When associated with atopy the prognosis also tends to be poor. Nail changes including pitting and distortion of the nail plate are sometimes seen in alopecia areata and this is more likely if the alopecia is extensive.

Trauma (Figure 10.5) to hair that is self-inflicted may be intentional or accidental. Thus pony tails, various racial hair styles, trendy styles, tight rollers and hot combs may cause patchy alopecia unintentionally. Head pressure and movement combine to produce the common temporary occipital hair loss seen in infants. Trichotillomania is the term sometimes used to describe the self-limiting form of alopecia produced either consciously, or involuntarily, as the result of habit. Thus, children may cause breakage of

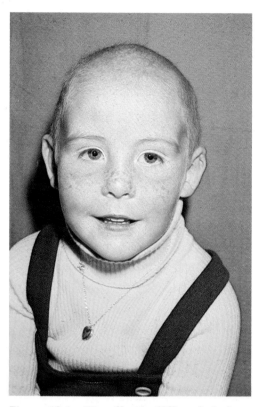

Figure 10.1   Hereditary diffuse hair loss
This child had scalp hypotrichosis as her only
abnormality.

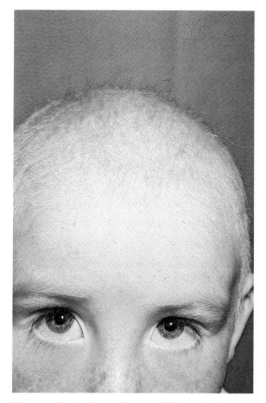

Figure 10.2   **Hereditary diffuse hair loss**
Close-up.

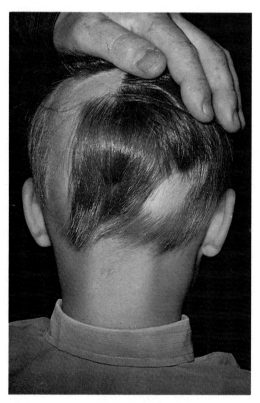

Figure 10.3   Alopecia areata   Excessive hair
loss is visible over posterior scalp.

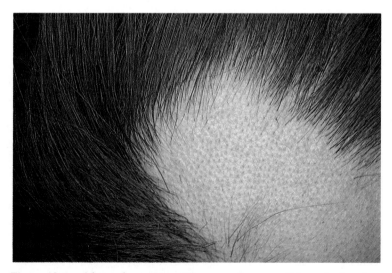

Figure 10.4   **Alopecia areata**   Close-up of an area of alopecia showing
exclamation mark hairs between 9 and 2 o'clock.

hairs by the common habit of twisting groups of hairs, or they can pull out or cut their own hair intentionally. Usually of no consequence, it can be important if persistent and extensive, posing a major threat to both child and family in terms of emotional stability. Clinically, differentiation from alopecia areata is usually based on the irregular outline, bizarre appearance and the presence of short stub-like hairs in trichotillomania. Sometimes scalp hair fall in children may result from others pulling out the hair.

Scarring alopecia (Figure 10.6)
This is the end result of a number of inflammatory processes resulting in irreversible scarring of the affected area. Local infections, trauma and various dermatoses may produce scarring. Aplasia cutis is a rare developmental deformity in some cases genetically determined, most commonly affecting the posterior scalp. A crust or ulcer present at birth heals leaving a scar.

Systemic disorders (Figures 10.7, 10.8) such as iron deficiency, hypopituitarism, hypothyroidism and hyperthyroidism may result in excessive hair fall. Telogen effluvium may follow severe mental or physical stress such as occurs with fever, meningitis, surgery or active colitis.

Drug alopecia will be seen particularly with cytotoxic drugs and anticoagulants which damage rapidly dividing cells in the hair bulb and root sheaths. This anagen effluvium is reversible. Transient hair loss may be seen with sodium valproate and when regrowth occurs hair may be more curly than normal.

Ringworm of the scalp (tinea capitis) is described in Chapter 5.

HAIR SHAFT DEFORMITIES
Monilethrix (beading of hair) (Figure 10.9) is an autosomal dominant condition which always affects scalp hairs producing partial alopecia but other hairs can be affected. Individual hairs show beading with the elliptical nodes 0·7–1 mm apart separated by narrow internodes at which the medulla is lacking. The internodes break transversely so that hair fails to grow to any appreciable length. The condition is permanent.

Pili torti (twisting of hair) (Figure 10.10) indicates multiple 180° twists each no more than a fraction of a millimetre long occurring with scalp hair particularly. It can occur alone as an isolated autosomal dominant inherited condition but may occur in other inherited syndromes. When light is shone on twisted hair at varying angles, a flickering or spangling effect is seen.

Trichorrhexis nodosa is a condition in which there is an inherent weakness of the hair shaft so that, with minor trauma such as brushing or shampooing, the shaft readily fractures through the centre of a node.

Woolly hair (Figure 10.11) may occur as a localized hair naevus, which is a developmental abnormality, or as an inherited condition in Caucasians affecting the whole scalp and giving the appearance of negroid hair. This latter condition is termed the *woolly hair syndrome* and although usually autosomal dominant it may be autosomal recessive. The onset is at birth with maximum severity in childhood when the curl diameter is

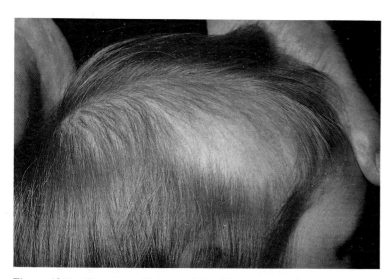

Figure 10.5   **Trauma**   Boy, aged 2, with traumatic alopecia right side of scalp.

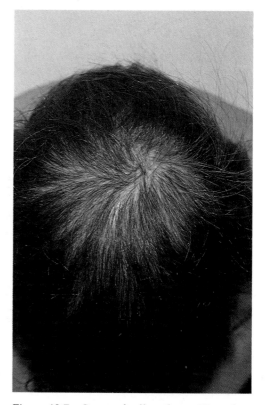

Figure 10.7   **Systemic disorders**   Hypothyroidism was the cause of hair fall in this child.

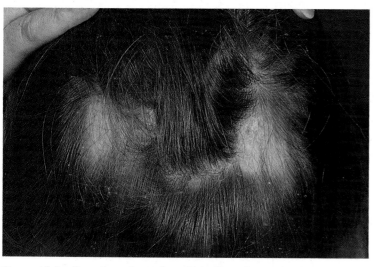

Figure 10.6   **Scarring alopecia**   Girl of 9 with two patches of scarring alopecia over anterior half of scalp. The mother was uncertain whether they were present at birth, but aplasia cutis is likely.

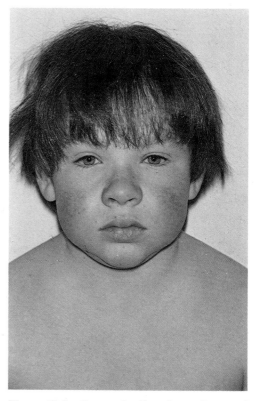

Figure 10.8   **Systemic disorders**   Facies of same child.

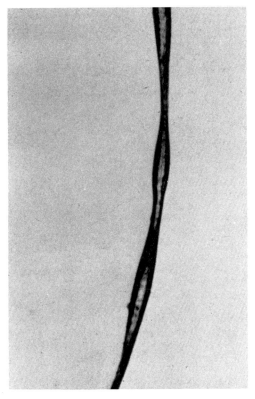

Figure 10.9 **Monilethrix** A magnified single hair with beading and narrow internodes is shown. (Courtesy of Dr R. Dawber)

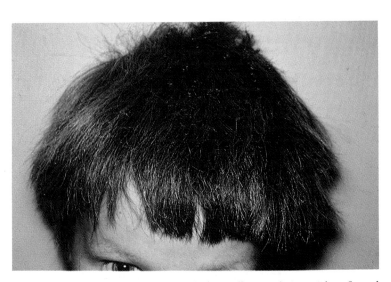

Figure 10.10 **Pili torti** The flickering effect on hairs with reflected light at the site of the twists is seen over the anterior scalp in the midline.

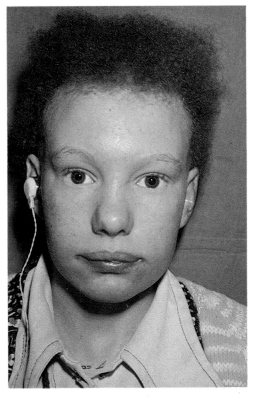

Figure 10.11 **Woolly hair** This white girl, aged 13, had the woolly hair syndrome. In addition, she had congenital perceptive deafness and ichthyosis vulgaris.

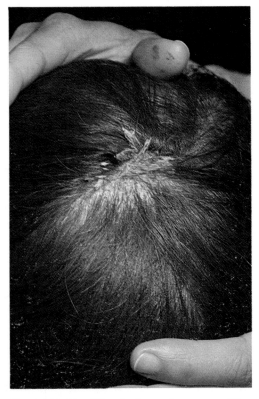

Figure 10.12 **Pityriasis amiantacea** The asbestos-like scales surrounding the proximal portion of the hair shaft are well shown.

approximately 0·5 cm and it is very difficult to brush or comb the woolly wiry hair. 180° axial rotation of the hair shaft is invariable and trichorrhexis nodosa is common.

PITYRIASIS AMIANTACEA (Figure 10.12) describes a not uncommon condition in which white asbestos-like scales cling firmly to the scalp hair shaft and extend some distance along them. Commonly, only a small area of scalp is affected. When the scales are removed hair may be removed with them, but the hair will usually regrow when the condition is effectively treated. It may occur *per se* but can also be an early stage of psoriasis.

Nails

CONGENITAL ABNORMALITIES

Nail–patella syndrome (Figures 10.13, 10.14) is an autosomal dominant condition characterized by small or rudimentary patellae, elbow joint deformities, and iliac spurs, in addition to abnormal nail formation and renal abnormalities presenting as chronic glomerulonephritis. Some nails may be missing, reduced in size, or split longitudinally; thumb and index finger nails are particularly affected.

Pachyonychia congenita (Figures 10.15, 10.16) is a rare autosomal dominant disorder in which the nails are abnormal from birth, later developing wedge-like thickening with exaggeration of the transverse curvature. Recurrent nail shedding can occur in infancy. Palmar and plantar hyperkeratosis occurs in childhood and oral leukoplakia frequently occurs in later childhood.

Koilonychia (Figure 10.17) is seen frequently as a normal finding in the first few months of life due to relatively thin and soft nail plate. However, a dominant inherited persistent form exists and iron deficiency anaemia is a further cause.

INFECTIONS

Chronic paronychia (Figure 10.18) is seen most commonly in thumb- or finger-suckers. A mixed flora is often found of bacteria and *Candida albicans*. Deformity of the nail is a common complication. Cure requires correction of the sucking habit although, of course, the infection should be treated.

Ringworm (dermatophyte) (Figure 10.19) infection of the nails is uncommon in childhood but it certainly does occur and it is well worth examining the feet of family members because the source will often be found. Big toe-nails are particularly affected, being thickened, irregular and white or yellowish in colour. Topical miconazole cream alone or sometimes in conjunction with oral griseofulvin for 6–18 months can be prescribed. Any affected adult contacts should be treated more vigorously.

TRAUMA

Nail–biting (Figure 10.20) is common. The best advice to the child is to stop it because nails attacked may become permanently dystrophic if the matrix is damaged. Periungual warts are common in nail-biters.

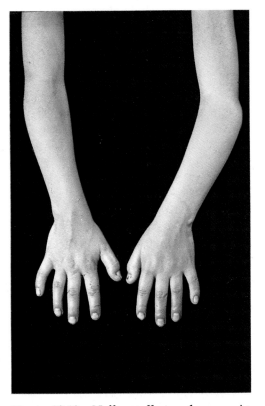

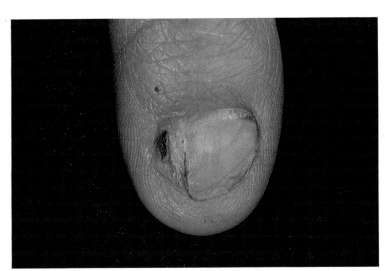

Figure 10.13 **Nail–patella syndrome** At left elbow the head of the radius is dislocated.

Figure 10.14 **Nail–patella syndrome** Close-up of partially absent right thumb-nail.

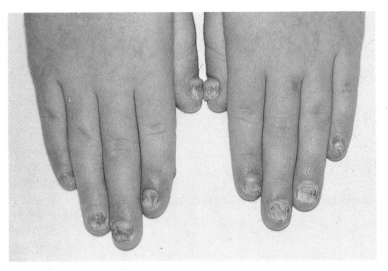

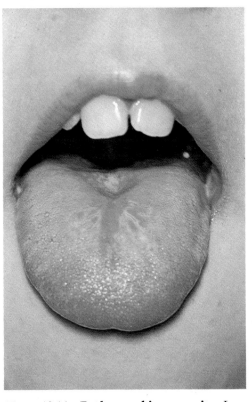

Figure 10.15 **Pachyonychia congenita** Child aged 7. Wedge appearance of thumb and right middle finger-nails is clearly shown.

Figure 10.16 **Pachyonychia congenita** Leukoplakia of tongue in same child.

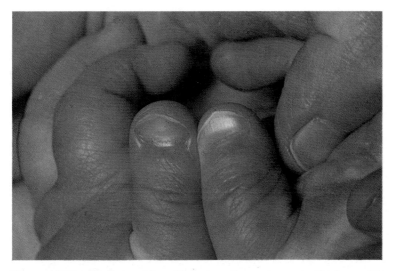

Figure 10.17   **Koilonychia**   Thumb-nails are shown in this boy of 2 but all 20 nails were affected.

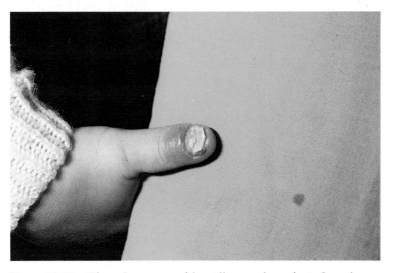

Figure 10.18   **Chronic paronychia**   Illustrated are the inflamed posterior nail fold and dystrophic nail in this thumb-sucker.

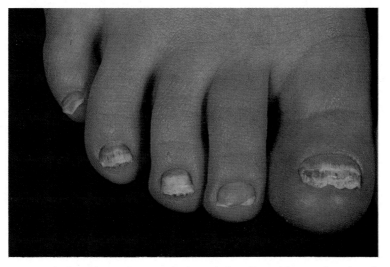

Figure 10.19   **Ringworm**   Thickened discoloured toe-nails infected with *T. rubrum* are shown in a boy of 3½ with abnormal nails since 8 months old. He received treatment with oral griseofulvin and topical miconazole.

Habit tic

A deformity consisting of a longitudinal depression down the centre of a nail, with numerous horizontal ridges extending across the nail from it, is caused by the patient picking at the cuticle or scratching the nail of the affected digit with a finger of the same hand. Usually the thumb-nail is affected. This condition differs from another of unknown cause termed median nail dystrophy.

Ingrowing toe-nail (Figures 10.21–10.23) is not uncommon in childhood contrary to popular belief. In infants a combination of walking and footwear pressure may induce pain, bacterial paronychia and overgrowth of granulation tissue around the soft pliable nail plate. In addition, incorrect cutting of the toe-nails is an important factor. However, a primary factor in infants can be unduly prominent skin at the extreme tip of the big toe forming an anterior nail fold which encourages ingrowing and prevents the free end of the big toe-nail growing normally; this condition may sometimes be genetically determined.

For ingrowing toe-nail local antiseptic measures will be required and advice to parents regarding avoidance of pressure trauma on the toes. Because of the likelihood of recurrence surgery should be avoided and where there is a prominent anterior nail fold this may spontaneously cease to overhang with time allowing normal nail growth.

Haemorrhage (Figure 10.24) under a nail may be due to obvious trauma, but high platform shoes and wedge heels worn by older children may not uncommonly cause haemorrhage under a nail and often separation of that nail.

BEAU'S LINES (Figures 10.25, 10.26) are transverse linear depressions of the nails which develop as a reaction to any severe illness or shock that temporarily interrupts nail formation. They become visible on the nail plate a few months after the onset of the disease that caused the condition. Since the lines originate under the proximal nail fold the date of the illness can be estimated by the distance of the depression from the cuticle.

TWENTY-NAIL DYSTROPHY (Figures 10.27, 10.28) is an idiopathic dystrophy, eventually of all 20 nails, that begins in early childhood. Excessive longitudinal ridging and opacity occurs. It tends to be self-limiting and reversible although any nail damage including atrophy or pterygium formation remains. Similar severe nail dystrophy is also seen in children in which ridging is not a prominent feature; koilonychia of thumb- and toe-nails may occur and some nails may be unaffected.

RIPPLED NAILS (Figure 10.29)

Distinct transverse rippling of the nails, giving an appearance likened to the sand after the tide has gone out, is seen occasionally. Of unknown cause its appearance is similar to the uniform pitting across the nail sometimes seen in psoriasis and alopecia areata.

GREAT TOE-NAIL DYSTROPHY (Figure 10.30)

It is not uncommon to see infants with developmentally abnormal toe-nails, particularly the big toe-nails, which are thickened and may show yellow to green discolouration. Often they are slow-growing or non-growing and they may be ridged transversely. Overcurvature in the long axis of the nail can produce in-growing in such a nail and will be encouraged by ill-fitting footwear.

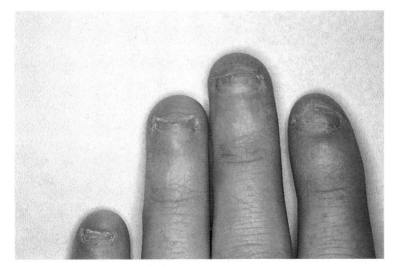

Figure 10.20 **Nail biting** Bitten finger nails.

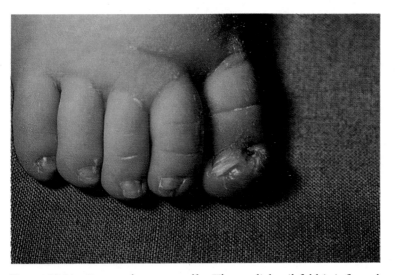

Figure 10.21 **Ingrowing toe-nail** The medial nail fold is inflamed here around the nail plate.

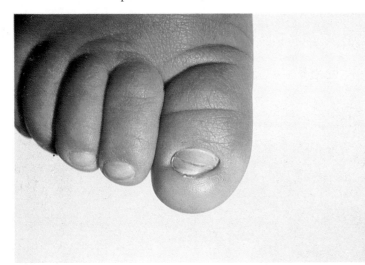

Figure 10.22 **Ingrowing toe-nail** Slowly growing big toe-nail in a child of 9 months.

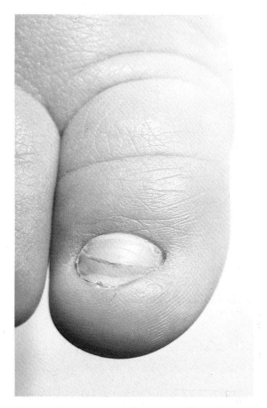

Figure 10.23 **Ingrowing toe–nail** Close-up of big toe in same child, showing an overhanging anterior nail fold. Inflammation began when he started wearing shoes at the age of 18 months. Soon after the age of 2 the toe tip ceased to overhang allowing the nail to grow normally.

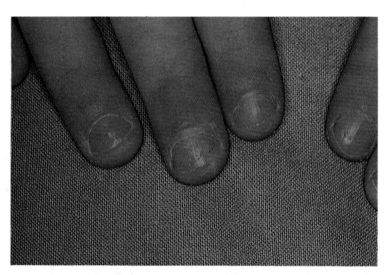

Figure 10.25 **Beau's lines** A transverse depression is visible over the distal half of all the nails.

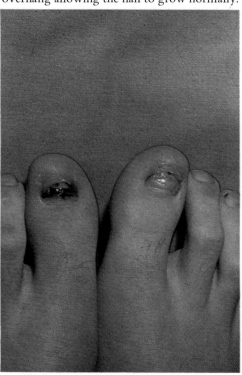

Figure 10.24 **Haemorrhage** Haemorrhage and loss of big toe–nails resulted from platform shoe trauma.

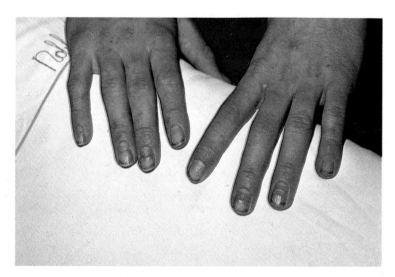

Figure 10.26 **Beau's lines** More marked example in which temporary shedding of the nails occurred. The boy had had infectious mononucleosis some months previously.

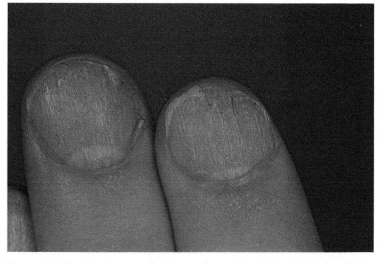

Figure 10.27 **Twenty–nail dystrophy** Close-up of ridged nails in a girl of 10.

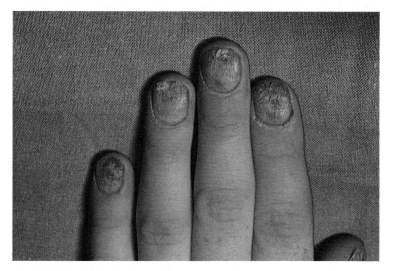

Figure 10.28 **Twenty-nail dystrophy** Thirteen–year-old boy showing severe nail dystrophy 2 years after onset. Note the ridged opaque nails and splitting of the free end of the nails. A further 3 years later there had been only minimal improvement.

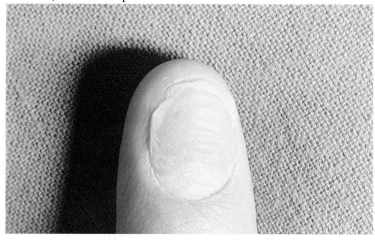

Figure 10.29 **Rippled nails** Girl of 12 with transverse pitting and ridging producing a rippled appearance to the nail. Many finger- and toe-nails were affected.

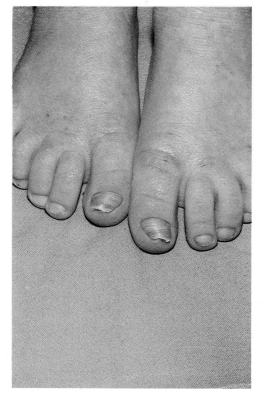

Figure 10.30 **Great toe-nail dystrophy** Thickened, ridged, discoloured, outwardly directed, incurved big toe-nails in a boy of 3½ years. They had never grown, the mother stated.

11

Trauma, drug eruptions, and miscellaneous

Trauma

SUNBURN (Figure 11.1) is defined as a cutaneous erythema of sufficient degree to cause discomfort, caused by sun exposure at wavelengths between 290 and 320 nm. Skin signs may vary from a mild erythema to a severe reaction with blister formation. Constitutional symptoms may be severe with extensive sunburn and include nausea, malaise, fever and delirium. Prophylactic measures are most important and this is particularly essential for infants and fair-skinned children who cannot tolerate sun exposure. Use of hats and long-sleeved clothing in addition to sunscreens are important and youngsters not used to regular sunlight exposure must not be exposed for too long a period, particularly during the peak ultraviolet exposure time between 10 a.m. and 2 p.m. Treatment of sunburn includes calamine lotion, and weak topical corticosteroids are also useful in severe acute cases.

SUBUNGUAL EXOSTOSIS (Figures 11.2, 11.3) is a solitary fibrous nodule on the terminal border of the distal phalanx of a toe or finger, particularly the big toe. Lesions may be due to trauma or occur spontaneously. They are not usually seen under the age of 4 years. A small flesh-coloured growth develops beneath, and projects sharply beyond the free edge of the nail often detaching the nail. It is often painful as it grows. Treatment of choice is excision by an orthopaedic surgeon.

PYOGENIC GRANULOMA (Figures 11.4, 11.5) is a vascular nodule which develops rapidly, often at the site of a recent injury. It is usually a dull-red fleshy polypoid lesion which may be pedunculated and easily bleeds with trauma. It may occur in any part of the mouth including the lips and other common sites are the fingers and upper trunk. The treatment is curettage, followed by cauterization or diathermy coagulation of the base. Many lesions recur with initial treatment and some may require excision.

BLACK HEEL (talon noir) (Figure 11.6) is a common asymptomatic condition occurring in athletic adolescents, particularly football and basketball players. Clusters of black specks appear at the back or side of the heel just above the hyperkeratotic edge of the

138

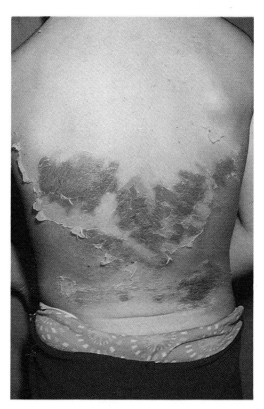

Figure 11.1 **Sunburn** Boy of 4 exposed to the sun for too long. An older sibling looking after him forgot about him.

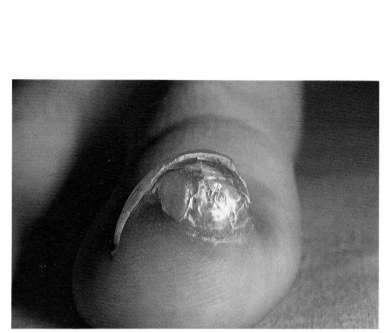

Figure 11.2 **Subungual exostosis** Note the lifted nail.

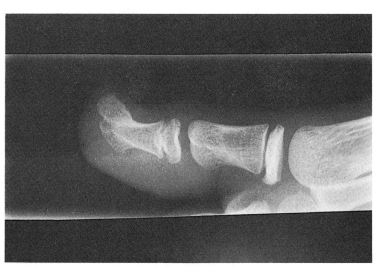

Figure 11.3 **Subungual exostosis** Radiograph of another patient.

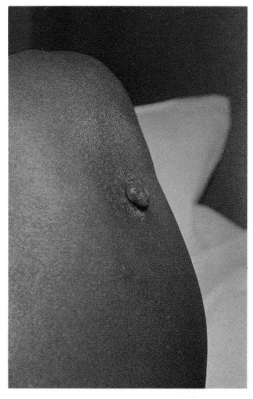

Figure 11.4 **Pyogenic granuloma** Girl of 10 with lesion over scapular region.

foot. The lesions resemble a tattoo and may be mistaken for plantar warts or even malignant melanoma. However, black heel tends to be bilateral and symmetrical. It is usually noted early on in the playing season and hardness of the ground seems relevant. In the disorder, papillary capillaries are ruptured by the shearing action associated with the sport.

DERMATITIS ARTEFACTA (Figure 11.7)
Very occasionally, a child is seen, usually an older girl, in whom deliberate self-mutilation of the skin is suspected. The resulting ulceration, excoriation, or purpura is bizarre in appearance and invariably accessible to self-infliction. Characteristically, occluded lesions heal rapidly only to recur with further exposure. It usually occurs in intellectually dull and unsophisticated children as a form of attention seeking or protest. Usually a histrionic gesture, most cases have no significance beyond a limited nuisance value. Rarely, early schizophrenia may present in this way in the adolescent.

TATTOOS (Figure 11.8) may be seen in older children who may prick particles of soot or Indian ink into the skin with any pointed object, or submit to tattooing under the influence of their companions. Some who submit are unstable and emotionally immature. Carbon is completely inert, but allergic sensitivity to cinnabar (affecting red areas) and chrome salts (affecting green areas) may occur. Frequently, removal of tattoos is requested on cosmetic or aesthetic grounds and simple excision is the treatment of choice for smaller lesions.

NON-ACCIDENTAL INJURY (Figure 11.9) may be visible in the skin as bruising, ulceration or hair loss and it is good practice to notice any signs of possible trauma when fully examining a child's skin. The family background will of course, be relevant, in suspected cases.

Drug eruptions

SCRATCH MARKS (Figure 11.10)
It should be remembered that pruritus may precede a drug eruption and in fact can occur without any rash ever appearing. Severe pruritus will be accompanied by scratching.

EXANTHEMATIC (Figures 11.11, 11.12)
This term indicates a widespread erythematous maculo-papular eruption which may be morbilliform. Ampicillin and phenytoin are common causes in children. Ampicillin eruptions are normally exanthematic and appear 5–14 days after starting treatment. Almost all patients with infectious mononucleosis given ampicillin early in the course of infection, develop a distinct irritant copper-coloured purpuric maculo-papular eruption over the trunk and then limbs, 7–10 days after starting antibiotic therapy; the same eruption may occur much less commonly with other pencillins.

URTICARIA of ordinary type, of which drugs are an important cause, is discussed in Chapter 7.

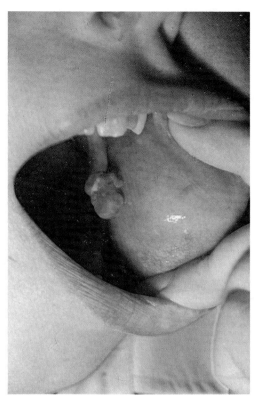

Figure 11.5 **Pyogenic granuloma** This lesion in a 12-year-old girl was treated with curette and cautery under local anaesthetic.

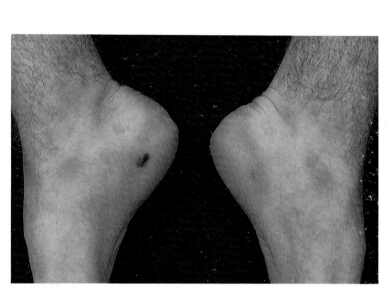

Figure 11.6 **Black heel** Note the bilateral symmetrical involvement of the heels.

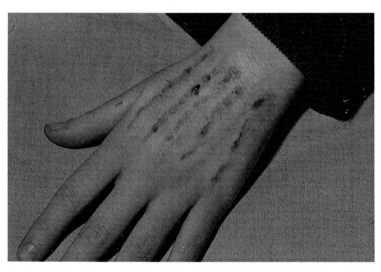

Figure 11.7 **Dermatitis artefacta** Typical bizarre appearance of lesions.

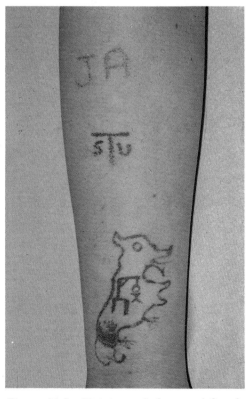

Figure 11.8 **Tattoos** A depressed female with self-inflicted lesions.

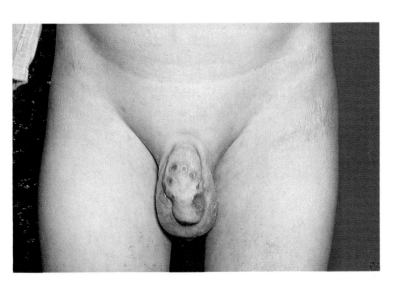

Figure 11.9 **Non-accidental injury** Penile burns produced by a cigarette.

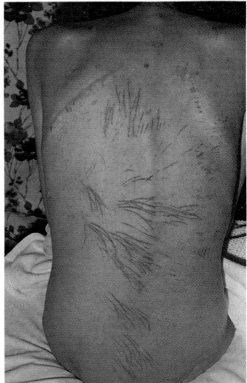

Figure 11.10 **Drug eruption** Scratch marks in a girl of 15 with intense itching. This preceded an exanthematic eruption due to a diuretic given in a high dosage for cardiac failure.

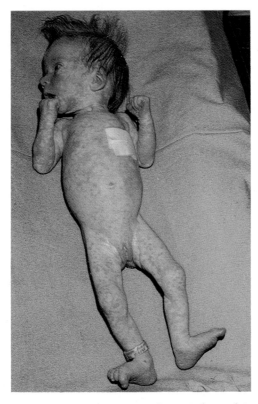

Figure 11.11 **Drug eruption** Infant of 2 months with exanthematic eruption due to amoxycillin.

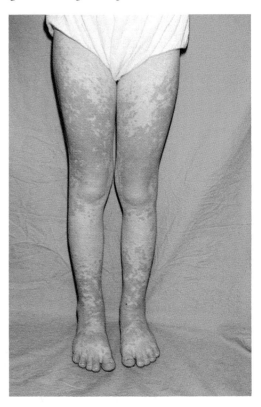

Figure 11.12 **Drug eruption** Girl of 6 with florid exanthem which was most marked over limbs. She had received amoxycillin, ampicillin and erythromycin, and ampicillin was considered the most likely cause.

CORTICOSTEROIDS (Figures 11.13–11.15)

Topical corticosteroids, particularly the more potent ones, can give rise to striae which are usually irreversible and skin atrophy which is often reversible. Both epidermal and dermal atrophy with increased skin fragility, telangiectasia, poikilodermatous change and loss of subcutaneous tissue can occur. Even small quantities of a steroid preparation stronger than hydrocortisone cream BPC or hydrocortisone ointment BP applied to the face for prolonged periods can produce marked skin atrophy. Excessive growth of hair is also occasionally seen at the site of prolonged steroid application, and infection is a not uncommon side-effect in view of the lowered resistance produced by steroid inhibition of the normal inflammatory response. Application, particularly under occlusion, of potent and usually fluorinated steroids, may lead to interference with pituitary–adrenal function and retard growth; this is of particular importance to note in infants.

Oral corticosteroids, administered on an intermittent basis, such as alternate days, are likely to cause significantly less growth retardation and somewhat less hypothalamic–pituitary–adrenal suppression than daily divided doses. Administration of supra-physiological doses of corticosteroids will result in the well-known clinical picture of Cushing's syndrome.

LAXATIVE ERUPTION (Figure 11.16)

Danthron is a synthetic anthraquinone compound contained in some laxative preparations. It can be converted to dithranol in the colon. It causes temporary and harmless pink-red coloration of urine and with prolonged regular use similar well-defined discoloration of skin in the perianal area, which may be seen in infants. If the drug is continued after the eruption has appeared, an irritant contact reaction can occur.

Miscellaneous

ACNE

Infantile acne (Figures 11.17–11.19) appears between the age of 3 or 4 months and 5 years. When acne does occur in children under 3 months of age it is sometimes referred to as acne neonatorum and it is commoner in boys. In the great majority of cases of infantile acne there is no evidence of endocrine disorder. Papules, pustules, nodules and cysts occur and there may be comedones. Most cases improve within a few years but some of these children tend to clear only to develop severe acne at adolescence. Treatment includes topical sulphur 1–3% in a cream or paste, although in more severe cases benzoyl peroxide preparations may be used. In view of the possibility of yellow or yellow-brown discoloration of deciduous or permanent teeth occurring with oral tetracyclines, these should be avoided not only in pregnancy and in infants but also in children up to the age of 12 years.

Acne vulgaris (Figures 11.20–11.22) in its mild form is so common that it may be considered physiological between the ages of 14 and 19. However, it can be severe and produce both physical and mental discomfort. Topical treatments include benzoyl peroxide and retinoic acid creams. It should be noted that adolescents between 14 and 17 appear to respond to acne treatment more slowly than older individuals.

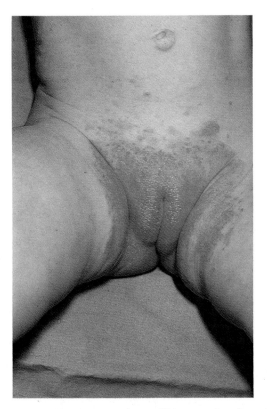

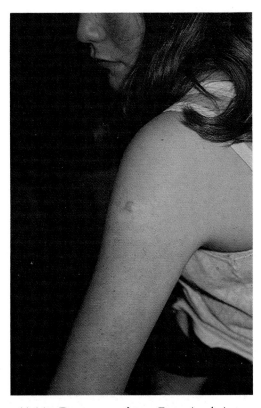

Figure 11.13 **Drug eruption** This eruption in a 21-month-old baby was due to repeated application of a potent steroid. Local side-effects may be marked over the napkin area with abuse of topical steroids and absorption producing iatrogenic Cushing's syndrome has been described.

Figure 11.14 **Drug eruption** Excessive hair growth at the exact site of application of flurandrenolone-impregnated transparent tape. Application was daily for 16 hours in 24 for about a month, in the treatment of post-BCG vaccination keloid.

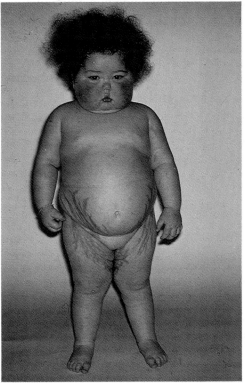

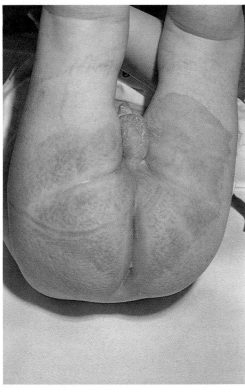

Figure 11.15 **Drug eruption** Gross Cushinoid appearance in a child treated with systemic corticosteroids for a haemolytic anaemia. Her appearance returned to normal after treatment.

Figure 11.16 **Drug eruption** Danthron eruption. Note the well-defined distribution where excreted drug has been spread by a soiled napkin.

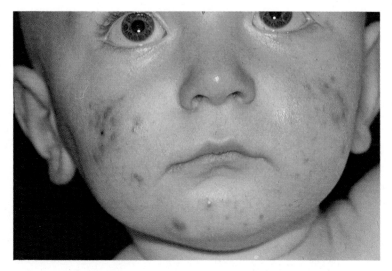

Figure 11.17 **Infantile acne** One-year-old boy, with pustules and papules over cheeks and chin.

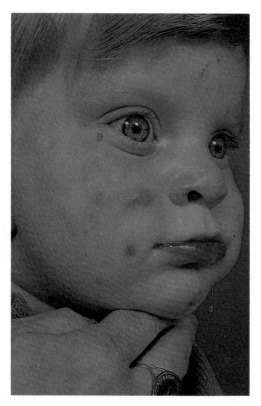

Figure 11.18 **Infantile acne** Another 1-year-old boy with florid cheek lesions.

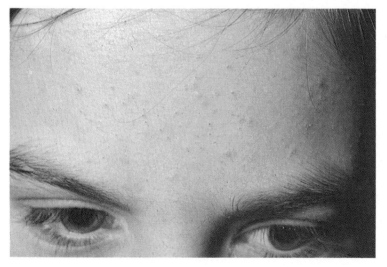

Figure 11.19 **Infantile acne** Showing yellow-brown tetracycline staining of deciduous teeth. (Courtesy of Dr W. R. Tyldesley)

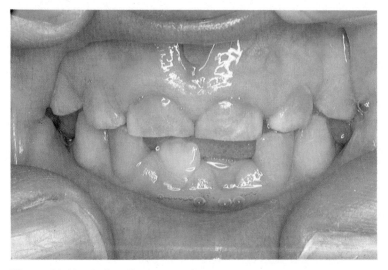

Figure 11.20 **Acne vulgaris** Blackheads are prominent over the forehead in this 12-year-old.

MILIA (Figure 11.23) which are small subepidermal keratin cysts are not only common in the newborn (see Chapter 3) but at all ages. Many arise in underdeveloped sebaceous glands or they can arise in damaged sweat ducts. The whitish lesions are usually noticed on the cheeks and eyelids, particularly at the sites of vellus hair follicles. Milia may also follow blister formation anywhere, as in dermolytic bullous dermatosis.

MOUTH

Scrotal tongue (Figure 11.24) is a developmental defect which in mild form is of common occurrence. It may present in infancy but may not manifest until later life. Clinically it has a deep longitudinal groove with more or less deep radiating grooves dividing the tongue into various configurations.

Erythema migrans (geographic tongue) (Figure 11.24) is a benign inflammatory disorder of unknown origin. Children under the age of 4 years are most commonly affected. It may be associated with a scrotal tongue but the latter usually develops later. Multiple smooth red patches on the dorsum of the tongue are outlined by a white, slightly elevated margin. The configuration of the patches, which are formed by desquamation of the filiform papillae, is constantly changing to form map-like patterns. There are usually no symptoms, but soreness particularly with hot foods or drinks, may occur.

White sponge naevus (white folded gingivostomatitis) (Figure 11.25) is a benign epithelial irregularity determined by an autosomal dominant gene. The lesions may be present at birth or appear during childhood or adolescence. The affected mucosa is white, thickened, folded and feels soft and spongy and the greater part of the buccal mucosa may be affected. Similar changes are sometimes found in the anal canal or vagina.

PIGMENTATION DISORDERS

Oculocutaneous albinism (Figure 11.26) results from failure of melanocytes in skin, hair and eye to synthesize normal amounts of melanin. The condition is inherited as an autosomal recessive trait. The skin colour is light and the hair whitish–yellow. The skin is very sensitive to solar radiation and in time solar changes, with the appearance of solar keratoses and skin carcinomata are common. There is also photophobia, reduced visual acuity and nystagmus.

Vitiligo (Figures 11.27, 11.28) is a common disorder said to occur in 1% of the world's population. In about half of the affected individuals it develops before the age of 20. The aetiology is unknown but between 30 and 40% of patients have a positive family history. There is a marked absence of melanocytes and melanin in the affected epidermis. Hypopigmented areas are first noted, usually on the sun exposed areas of skin of the backs of hands. Lesions then become more widespread and usually symmetrical in distribution. However, sometimes vitiligo is unilateral and may have a dermatomal (segmental) arrangement. Vitiliginous areas are prone to sunburn. The white macules have a convex outline, increase irregularly in size, and fuse with neighbouring lesions. In older lesions hairs are often white. Margins of lesions may become hyperpigmented particularly after sun exposure. The condition is gradually progressive. Spontaneous repigmentation occurs in about 10% of patients but is usually only partial. Vitiligo is

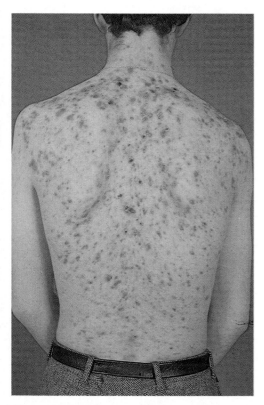

Figure 11.21 **Acne vulgaris** Severe widespread inflammatory lesions in this boy.

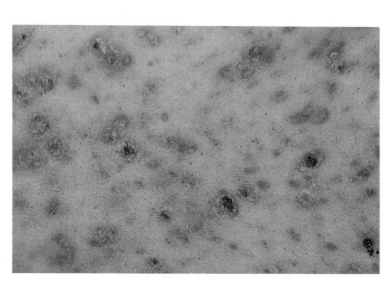

Figure 11.22 **Acne vulgaris** Close-up.

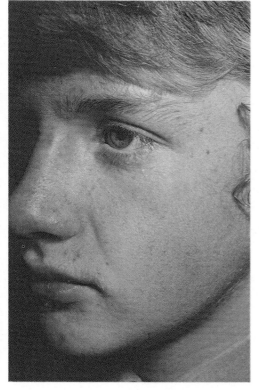

Figure 11.23 **Milia** Note the white papules under the left eye. He was not concerned about his mild acne over the nose and chin.

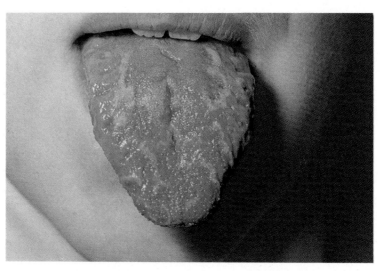

Figure 11.24 **Scrotal tongue and erythema migrans** This boy of 10 demonstrates both a scrotal tongue and erythema migrans. Note the white elevated margin outlining the smooth migratory patches.

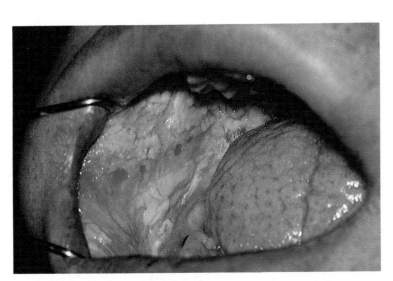

Figure 11.25 **White sponge naevus** The spongy patches over the buccal mucosa are well-shown.

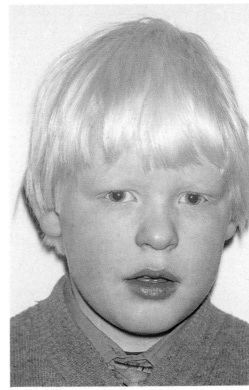

Figure 11.26 **Oculocutaneous albinism** Boy of 8 showing white hair, white eyebrows and white eyelashes. The pupils appear red even in normal daylight since light enters the eye not only through the pupil but also through the iris and sclera. (Courtesy of Mr J. S. Cant)

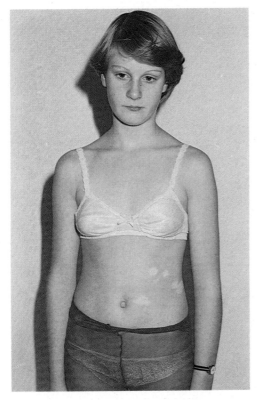

Figure 11.27 **Vitiligo** This girl of 14 shows unilateral localized segmental vitiligo.

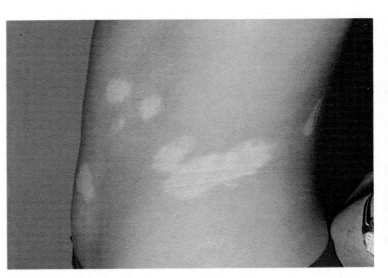

Figure 11.28 **Vitiligo** Close-up of affected area.

associated with a number of disorders considered to be auto-immune and halo naevi may antedate the onset of vitiligo.

Naevus anaemicus (Figure 11.29) is a developmental abnormality characterized by a circumscribed round or oval patch of pale skin. The pallor of the naevus is due at least in part to increased sensitivity of the vessels to circulating catecholamines. It may occur on any part of the body but is usually seen on the trunk. It may be present at birth or appear in early childhood.

Erythema dyschromicum perstans (ashy dermatosis) (Figures 11.30–11.32) was first described in 1957 in El Salvador. Most cases have come from Central, North and South America. It is a chronic disease of unknown aetiology but without systemic effects. Sex incidence is equal and it usually presents in early adult life but children over the age of 5 years can be affected. Widespread asymptomatic or slightly irritant slaty-grey macules or plaques appear over trunk and limbs and active lesions may show a raised edge. Histologically the active border of the lesions shows hydropic degeneration of the basal layer with pigmentary incontinence. Although chronic, the condition does show a tendency to resolve in some children.

KWASHIORKOR (Figures 11.33, 11.34) seen in starving children is produced by severe protein deficiency and is characterized by localized or generalized oedema, apathy, anorexia, growth retardation, diarrhoea and skin changes. The condition most affects children from 4 months to 4 years of age and the most striking skin manifestation is hyperpigmented scaly plaques, especially prominent on the limbs. They peel leaving hypopigmented macules. Chronic pellagra lesions in contrast are localized to light-exposed areas. Apart from the plaques, the skin is generally dry and atrophic. Diffuse hair loss, haemorrhagic blisters, large areas of erosion, and secondary bacterial infection also occur. Treatment of the dry skin is with emollients, and infection should also be treated. However, correction of the underlying malnutrition is the main priority in treatment. It should be noted that kwashiorkor can also occur in malnourished children in an affluent society.

ATROPHIC CONDITIONS
Granuloma annulare (Figures 11.35, 11.36) which is of unknown cause is characterized by asymptomatic papules grouped in a ring-like distribution. It may occur anywhere but is most common over bony prominences and particularly over the hands and feet. Children and young adults are most commonly affected and it is more common in females. Early lesions begin as smooth flesh-coloured papules that slowly undergo central involution and peripheral extension to form oval or irregular rings with elevated often beaded borders. Lesions may be single or multiple and are usually 1–3 cm in diameter but more extensive patches, sometimes with a somewhat violaceous hue, may occur. Deeper subcutaneous lesions are also seen. Lesions tend to disappear spontaneously and attempts at treatment are unrewarding. However, some respond to topical and intralesional steroids.

Necrobiosis lipoidica (Figures 11.37, 11.38) is a degenerative disorder of dermal connective tissue, seen particularly in diabetics; it may also precede the onset of diabetes by a few years. The disorder may occur at any age. Lesions are most common over the

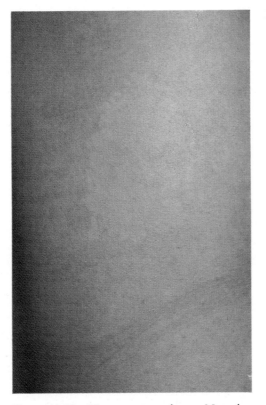

Figure 11.29 **Naevus anaemicus** Note the pale oval patch with a somewhat irregular edge, in an area of normal skin.

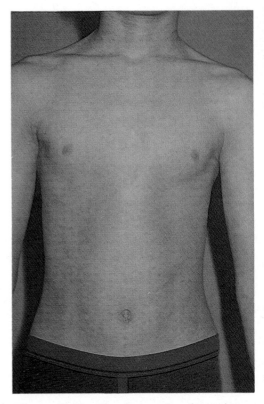

Figure 11.30 **Erythema dyschromicum perstans** Widespread eruption in a dark-skinned boy of 13.

Figure 11.31 **Erythema dyschromicum perstans** Close-up of slaty-grey macules.

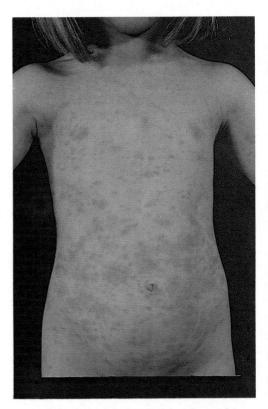

Figure 11.32 **Erythema dyschromicum perstans** White-skinned girl of 6 showing pigmented macules of different sizes over the trunk.

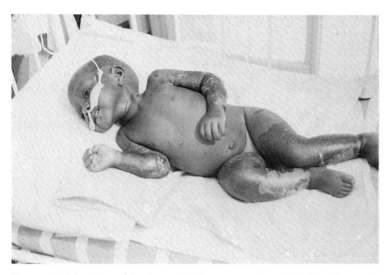

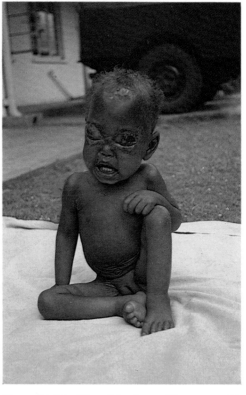

Figure 11.33 **Kwashiorkor** Eighteen-month-old infant from the Gambia showing hyperpigmented plaques over limbs and some hypopigmented areas. (Courtesy of Professor R. G. Hendrickse)

Figure 11.34 **Kwashiorkor** Two-year-old child with ulcerated skin over face. (Courtesy of Professor R. G. Hendrickse)

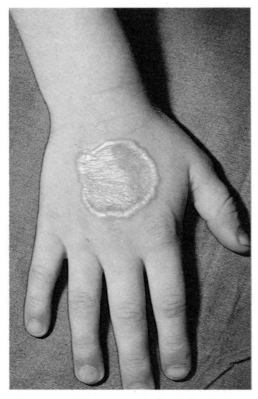

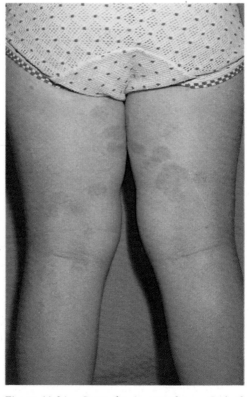

Figure 11.35 **Granuloma annulare** Typical smooth, ringed patch with raised edge. (Courtesy of Dr A. Lyell)

Figure 11.36 **Granuloma annulare** Girl of $2\frac{1}{2}$ years with large violaceous patches of granuloma annulare over posterior thighs.

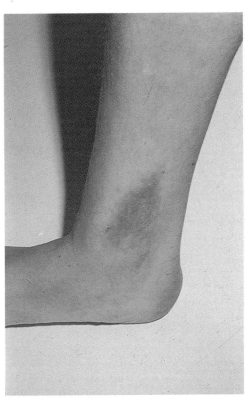

Figure 11.37 **Necrobiosis lipoidica**   Red-brown ankle plaque in a diabetic girl of 12.

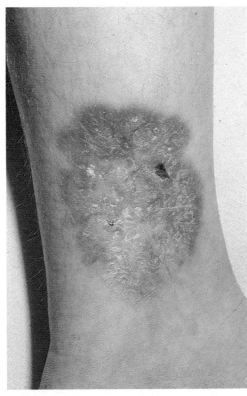

Figure 11.38 **Necrobiosis lipoidica**   Close-up of same region 3½ years later with outer portion showing telangiectasia, and yellow colour due probably to carotene. Two years before this photograph was taken, the central portion of the necrobiotic patch had ulcerated and the ulcerated area was excised and a skin graft applied.

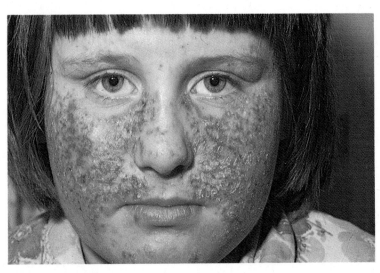

Figure 11.39 **Hutchinson's summer prurigo**   Severe eczematization in a young girl.

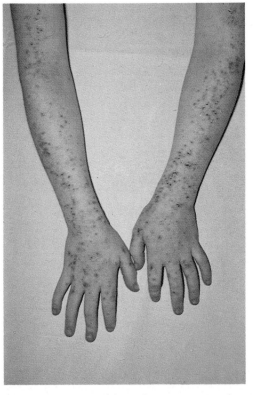

Figure 11.40 **Hutchinson's summer prurigo** Same girl. Eczematous papules over exposed upper limbs.

pretibial areas and they begin as an erythematous papule or patch which gradually enlarges and develops slowly into a brownish-yellow sclerotic plaque. The centre of the plaque is often atrophic with a translucent surface. Treatment of the lesions is unsatisfactory and they are often best left untreated. Early lesions can sometimes be aborted with intralesional triamcinolone but this may produce ulceration in older lesions. Spontaneous ulceration of lesions is best treated with local applications, although extensive ulceration may benefit from excision and full thickness grafting of the ulcerated area.

PHOTODERMATOSES

Polymorphic light eruption may start in early childhood but usually first appears in early adult life. It is sometimes familial and is more common in females. Multiple small itchy red papules which may become confluent occur on exposed areas, in the summer season. In many patients there is a delay of several hours to a few days between sun exposure and the onset of the eruption. There is a tendency for the eruption to be less severe as the summer progresses in a particular patient. Short wavelength ultraviolet light 290–320 nm is always involved, but longer wavelengths may also be relevant in some patients.

Hutchinson's summer prurigo (actinic prurigo) (Figures 11.39, 11.40) is a similar condition, again more common in females with an onset in childhood usually before puberty, in which persistent irritant papules occur not only on exposed sites but often on covered areas also. The papules are often excoriated showing weeping and crusting. In some cases it may be present all the year round but with worsening in summer. Prognosis is variable but many children clear after a period of years. A familial form of the disorder occurs in North American Indians. Management includes advice on suitable clothing and use of sunscreening agents.

Some other photodermatoses are mentioned in Chapter 2 and elsewhere.

Index

All numbers are page numbers—those in **bold face** refer to illustrations

acne   143
  infantile   143, **145**
  vulgaris   143, **145**, **147**
acrodermatitis enteropathica   32, **34**
acropustulosis of infancy   93, **96**, 97
actinic prurigo   *see* Hutchinson's summer prurigo
alopecia   126
  areata   26, 126, **127**
    nails   126, 134
  drug   128
  hereditary diffuse   126, **127**
  ringworm   81, **82**, **83**
  scarring   128, **129**
  systemic disorders   128, **129**
  traumatic   126, 128, **129**
anagen effluvium   128
angiofibromata   32, **33**
angioma serpiginosum   20, **21**
aplasia cutis   128, **129**
ashy dermatosis   *see* erythema dyschromicum
    perstans
atopic dermatitis   56–64
  eczema herpeticum   **63**
  eyelids   **61**
  follicular papules   62, **63**
  increased palmar markings   **60**
  infected   **58**, **59**
  infraorbital creases   **61**
  keratosis pilaris   **61**
  knee involvement   **60**
  lichenification   **59**
  lips   **62**
  pityriasis alba   **62**
  sparing napkin area   **57**
  treatment   64
  white dermographism   **63**
auricular appendage   10, **11**

Beau's lines   134, **136**
black heel   138, **141**
Bloch–Sulzberger syndrome   *see* incontinentia
    pigmenti

blue naevus   12
  cellular   **14**
  ordinary   **13**
bullous dermatoses   118–25
bullous ichthyosiform erythroderma
    see epidermolytic hyperkeratosis
bullous impetigo   **53**, 55
bullous pemphigoid   **124**, 125

café-au-lait patches   10, **13**, 28, **31**
calcinosis cutis   116, **117**
candidiasis   78
  in newborn   44, 50, **51**
cavernous haemangioma   16, **19**, **21**
cayenne pepper spots   **106**
cellulitis   70, **73**
chilblains   104, **107**, **108**
chronic bullous dermatosis of childhood   120,
    122, **123**
chronic paronychia   131, **133**
chronic pellagra   149
Chyletiella species   81
Cockayne's disease   118, **119**
collodion baby   32, **35**, 40, **43**, **45**
comedone naevus   **23**, 24
compound naevus   12, **14**
congenital lymphoedema   10, **11**
congenital syphilis   **53**, 55
connective tissue disorders   110–17
contact dermatitis   66
  irritant   **68**
  allergic   **68**
corticosteroids, dangers of   143, **144**
creeping eruption   86, **87**
Cushing's syndrome, iatrogenic   143, **144**
cutaneous larva migrans   *see* creeping eruption
cutaneous leishmaniasis   **86**, 87
cutis marmorata   40, **41**

dermatitis artefacta   140, **141**
dermatitis herpetiformis   120, **124**
dermatomyositis   113, **114**

dermolytic bullous dermatosis   120
  autosomal dominant   **121**
  autosomal recessive   **122**
    syndactyly   **122**
developmental abnormalities   10–25
diaper dermatitis   *see* napkin dermatitis
diffuse palmoplantar keratoderma   *see* tylosis
Down's syndrome   26
drug eruptions   140
  corticosteroids   143, **144**
  exanthematic   **142**
  laxative   143, **144**
  scratch marks   **142**
  urticaria   100
dyshidrotic eczema   *see* pompholyx
dystrophic epidermolysis bullosa   *see* dermolytic
    bullous dermatosis

ecthyma   70, **72**
ectodermal dysplasia
  anhidrotic   **38, 39**, 39
  hidrotic   26, **27**
eczema herpeticum   **63**, 64
Ehlers–Danlos syndrome   27, 28, **29**
epidermolysis bullosa   118
  hereditaria letalis (Herlitz)   118
  recurrent bullous eruption of hands and feet
    (Cockayne)   **119**
  simplex   **119**
epidermolytic hyperkeratosis   20, 28, **30, 31**
erysipelas   *see* cellulitis
erythema
  annulare centrifugum   100, **101**
  dyschromicum perstans   149, **150**
  infectiosum   78, **80**
  marginatum   **115**, 116
  migrans   146, **147**
  multiforme   98, **99**
  nodosum   98, **99**
  toxic   98, **101**
  toxic, of the newborn   40, **41**
erythropoietic protoporphyria   28, **29**

faun-tail naevus   **23**, 24
flea bites   **85**, 87
focal dermal hypoplasia   36, **37, 38**
freckles (ephelides)   10, **11**
frictional lichenoid dermatitis   64, **65**

genodermatoses   26–39
geographic tongue   *see* mouth, erythema migrans
giant pigmented naevus   12, **15**
Goltz syndrome   *see* focal dermal hypoplasia
granuloma annulare   149, **151**
great toenail dystrophy   134, **137**

habit tic   134
haemangioma   16
haemorrhage under nail   134, **136**
hair   126–31

hair shaft deformities   128
  monilethrix   **130**
  pili torti   **130**
  trichorrhexis nodosa   128, 131
  woolly hair   **130**
halo naevus   12, **15**, 149
hand, foot and mouth disease   78, **80**
hereditary diffuse hair loss   126, **127**
herpes
  simplex   74
    eczema herpeticum   *see* atopic dermatitis
    neonatal infection   74
    secondary   **77**
    stomatitis   **76, 77**
    vulvo-vaginitis   **76**
  zoster   **77**, 78
Hutchinson's summer prurigo   **152**, 153
hypertrophic scar   116, **117**
hypotrichosis   *see* hereditary diffuse hair loss

ichthyosis   28, 32, 39
  epidermolytic hyperkeratosis   **30, 31**
  lamellar   **35**
  non-bullous ichthyosiform erythroderma   **34**
  vulgaris   **29, 30**, 56
  X-linked   **39**
impetigo   70, **71, 72**
  in newborn   **53, 55**
incontinentia pigmenti   36, **38**
increased palmar markings   28, **30**, 56, **60**
infantile gluteal granuloma   44, **47**
infantile seborrhoeic dermatitis   44, **48, 49**
  erythroderma in   44
infections
  bacterial   70, **71–3**
  fungal   78, **80, 82, 83**
  viral   **73**, 74, **75–7**
infections and infestations   70–87
infectious mononucleosis   140
infestations   81, **83–6**
inflamed linear epidermal naevus   20, **23**
ingrowing toenail   134, **135, 136**
insect bites   **85**, 87
intertrigo   50, **52**
intradermal naevus   12, **14**
irritant napkin dermatitis   *see* napkin dermatitis

junctional bullous epidermatosis   *see* epidermolysis
    bullosa, hereditaria letalis
junctional naevus   12, **14**
juvenile melanoma   **15, 16, 17**
juvenile plantar dermatosis   63, 64, **65**
juvenile xanthogranuloma   20, **22**

Kasabach–Merritt syndrome   16
keloid   116, **117**
keratosis pilaris   56, **61**
kerion   81, **83**
Koebner phenomenon   **75**, 88, **89**
koilonychia   131, **133**
kwashiorkor   149, **151**

Letterer–Siwe disease   **54**, 55
lice infestation   81, **85**
    treatment   87
lichenification   56, **59**
lichen planus   93, **96**
    lichen nitidus   93
lichen sclerosus et atrophicus   110, **112**
lichen striatus   66, **67**, **68**
linear IgA dermatosis of childhood   *see* chronic
        bullous dermatosis of childhood
livedo reticularis   113, **115**
lupus erythematosus   113
    systemic   **114**
lymphangioma circumscriptum   20, **21**

mast cell disease   *see* mastocytosis
mastocytosis   100, 104
    diffuse cutaneous form   100
        mast cell naevi   **103**
        urticaria pigmentosa   **102**, **103**
measles   78, **79**, **80**
melanocytic naevus   12, **14**, **15**, **17**
meningococcaemia   **73**, 74
Microsporum canis
    hair fluorescence   81, **82**
milia   146
    ordinary   **147**
    in newborn   40, **41**
miliaria   40, **42**, 44
molluscum contagiosum   74, **76**
Mongolian patches   10, **13**
monilethrix   128, **130**
morphoea   110
    common form   **111**
    linear   **111**
mouth   146
    erythema migrans   **147**
    scrotal tongue   **147**
    white sponge naevus   **148**

naevi   10–24
    dermal   **17–19**, **21**, 22
    epithelial   **22**, **23**
    pigmented   **11**, **13–15**, **17**
naevus
    anaemicus   149, **150**
    flammeus   *see* port-wine stain
    naevus-cell   *see* melanocytic naevus
    spilus   12, **15**
nail biting   131, **135**
nail–patella syndrome   131, **132**
nails   131–7
napkin area eruptions   44
napkin dermatitis   44, **45**, **46**, **47**
napkin psoriasis   44, **49**
necrobiosis lipoidica   149, **152**, 153
    ulceration   153
neurofibromatosis   10, 28, **31**
newborn   40–55
nits   81, **85**

non-accidental injury   12. **105**, 140, **142**
non-bullous ichthyosiform erythroderma   32, **34**
nummular eczema   **65**, 66

oculocutaneous albinism   146, **148**
oriental sore   *see* cutaneous leishmaniasis

pachyonychia congenita   131, **132**
papular urticaria   **85**, **86**, 87
perianal dermatitis   50, **52**
perniosis   *see* chilblains
Peutz–Jehgers syndrome   28, **31**
photodermatoses   **152**, 153
pigmentation disorders   146, **148**, **150**
pili torti   128, **130**
pityriasis
    alba   **62**, 64
    amiantacea   **130**, 131
    lichenoides   93, **95**
    rosea   93, **94**
    rubra pilaris   93, **95**, **96**
poikiloderma congenitale
        see Rothmund–Thomson syndrome
polyarteritis nodosa   113
    cutaneous   **115**
    systemic   113
polymorphic light eruption   153
pompholyx   64, **65**
port-wine stain   16, **17**, **18**
progressive systemic sclerosis   110, **112**
    nail fold telangiectasia   **112**
pseudoxanthoma elasticum   **35**, 36
psoriasis   88–92
    guttate   **89**
    in newborn   **49**, 50, **51**
    Koebner phenomenon in   **89**
    onycholysis   **91**
    plaque   **89–92**
    Woronoff ring   **90**
    treatment   88, **92**
purpura   104
    Henoch–Schönlein   **103**, **105**
    idiopathic thrombocytopenic   **105**
    pigmented purpuric dermatosis   **106**
pyogenic granuloma   138, **139**, **141**

Raynaud's
    disease   108, **108**
    phenomenon   108, 110
rheumatic fever   **115**, 116
rheumatoid arthritis
    Still's disease   **115**, 116
    juvenile   116
ringworm infection   81, 131
    body   **83**
    foot   **80**
    nail   **133**
    scalp   **82**, **83**, 128
rippled nails   134, **137**
Rothmund–Thomson syndrome   **35**, 36, **37**

salmon patches   16, **17**
scabies   50, 81
  human   **83, 84, 85**
    in newborn   **51**
      treatment   50
    animal   81
scleroderma   110, **111, 112**
scratch marks   *see* drug eruptions
scrotal tongue   26, 146, **147**
sebaceous gland hyperplasia   40, **42**
sebaceous naevus   **23**, 24
seborrhoeic dermatitis
  infantile   44, **48, 49**
  pubertal   66
    blepharitis   66, **67**
    dandruff   66
    otitis externa   **67**
slapped cheek   *see* erythema infectiosum
spider telangiectases   20, **21**
spindle-cell naevus   *see* juvenile melanoma
staphylococcal scalded skin syndrome   50, **52, 53**, 70, **71**
Stevens–Johnson syndrome   *see* erythema multiforme
Still's disease   *see* rheumatoid arthritis
Sturge–Weber syndrome   16
striae atrophicae   116, **117**
strawberry mark   16, **18, 19**
strawberry–cavernous haemangioma   16, **19, 21**
subungual exostosis   138, **139**
sunburn   138, **139**
superficial haemangioma   *see* strawberry mark
supernumerary nipple   10, **11**
Sutton's naevus   *see* halo naevus

talon noir   *see* black heel
tattoos   140, **141**
telogen effluvium   128
tetracycline teeth staining   143, **145**
thumb sucking   *see* chronic paronychia
toxic erythema   98, **101**
toxic erythema of the newborn   40, **41**
Touton giant cells   *see* juvenile xanthogranuloma

trauma   138–42
  nail   131, **135, 136**
Trichophyton
  rubrum   **133**
  verrucosum   81, **83**
  violaceum   **83**
trichorrhexis nodosa   *see* hair shaft abnormalities
trichotillomania   126
tuberous sclerosis   32, **33**
Turner's syndrome   26, **27**
  webbing of neck   **27**
twenty nail dystrophy   134, **137**
tylosis   32, **33**

urticaria   100
  ordinary   **101, 102**, 140
  physical
    cholinergic   100
    cold   100
    dermographism   **102**
      white   **63**, 64
urticaria pigmentosa   100, **102, 103**, 104

varicella   78, **79**
vascular disorders   98–109
verrucous naevus   20
  localized   **22**
  widespread   **22**
vitiligo   146
  halo naevi and   12, 149
  segmental   **148**

warts   **73**, 74, **75**, 131
white dermographism   **63**, 64
white sponge naevus   146, **148**
woolly hair   128
  naevus   128
  syndrome   **130**

xeroderma pigmentosum   36, **37**

zinc deficiency   32, **34**